Magnet Status

Assessing, Pursuing, and Achieving Nursing Excellence

Marian C. Turkel, RN, PhD

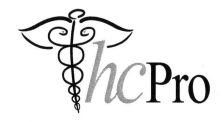

Marian C. Turkel, RN, PhD, Author

Susan H. Nick, RN, PhD, Contributing Author

John Gettings, Managing Editor

Naomi Funkhouser, Editorial Assistant

Lauren Rubenzahl, Copy Editor

Jean St. Pierre, Creative Director

Mike Mirabello, Senior Graphic Artist

Crystal Beland, Layout Artist

Susan Darbyshire, Cover Designer

Emily Sheahan, Executive Editor

Kathy Levesque, Group Publisher

Suzanne Perney, Publisher

Advice given is general. Readers should consult professional counsel for specific legal, ethical, or clinical questions.

Arrangements can be made for quantity discounts.

For more information, contact:

HCPro, Inc.
200 Hoods Lane
P.O. Box 1168
Marblehead, MA 01945
Telephone: 800/650-6787 or 781/639-1872
Fax: 781/639-2982
E-mail: *customerservice@hcpro.com*

Visit HCPro at its World Wide Web sites: *www.hcmarketplace.com* and *www.hcpro.com*

09/2004
20084

Contents

List of Figures

About the author

Marian C. Turkel, RN, PhD

Marian C. Turkel, RN, PhD, is an experienced nurse administrator, educator, researcher, and consultant. Dr. Turkel has been the coprincipal investigator on four federally funded research grants totaling almost $1,000,000. These research studies focused on organizational caring, nursing economics, nursing practice models, and workforce redevelopment. She has authored and coauthored multiple book chapters and articles in peer-reviewed nursing journals and has presented at both national and international conferences.

Dr. Turkel earned her PhD in nursing from the University of Miami and her Masters in Nursing Administration from Florida Atlantic University. Prior to relocating to Chicago from Miami Beach, FL, she was an assistant professor in the College of Nursing at Florida Atlantic University and taught courses in nursing leadership, research, healthcare economics, and caring theory at both the undergraduate and graduate levels. During this time, her interest in Magnet evolved, as she created her research initiatives, assisted graduate students working on projects to help their organizations obtain Magnet, and served as an external reviewer for hospitals pursuing Magnet status.

She is currently working as the Magnet project consultant at Northwestern Memorial Hospital in Chicago. Dr. Turkel is an adjunct faculty member in the Department of Public Health, Mental Health, and Administrative Nursing at the University of Illinois at Chicago, where she is involved in research initiatives looking at nursing practice in relation to healthcare labor force policy. She also maintains an independent consulting practice and is currently assisting a hospital in Florida as it pursues Magnet status.

Acknowledgments

A special thanks to my husband and soulmate, Brooks, for his ongoing love and caring energy. He has been my inspiration and is always there for me as I pursue my passions and scholarship. Thanks again for understanding why I didn't finish decorating the condo this summer, for eating leftovers, and for awakening my creative spirit through reflective dialogue at Oak Street beach on the weekends.

Thanks to my friend, mentor, guide, and colleague, Dr. Marilyn Ray. Early in my career, you had confidence in my ability to publish and do research, and this gave me the inner strength to pursue my doctorate. I would like to give a special acknowledgement to your husband Jim. We never would have come this far without his perseverance as he typed our first grant application.

Sincere thanks to Dr. Noreen Sugrue, my friend and colleague at the University of Illinois, for providing me with an opportunity to expand my research focus into the area of healthcare labor force policy. Thanks for having confidence and trust in me as we pursue our research journey.

Thanks to my friends and colleagues at Northwestern Memorial Hospital for the privilege of being a part of your Magnet journey.

Thanks to John and Naomi at HCPro for keeping me focused on the timeline and providing valuable editorial assistance. The book would not have happened if we hadn't developed a strong working relationship grounded in trust and mutual respect.

Thanks to my typist, Edna, for turning the chapters around on a tight timeline.

A special thanks to Dr. Susan Nick for writing Chapter 10, "Integration of nursing research." Your experience as a chief nurse executive came through as you discussed strategies for evidence-based practice within the reality of practice environments.

A very special acknowledgment to the dedication and commitment of all the chief nurse executives who have been instrumental in having their organizations achieve Magnet status. An additional thanks to those of you who were willing to share your experiences and stories. Your contributions were grounded in the realities of practice and will be helpful to your colleagues as they embark on the Magnet journey.

List of contributors

The following individuals contributed ideas, advice, and practice examples throughout this book. Please refer to this list for their titles and the names of their facilities.

- Janet Ahlstrom, MSN, RN, BC, M-SCNS, director of professional practice and nursing outcomes, Carondelet Health, Kansas City, MO

- Janet Cahill, RN, BSN, MBA, director of professional practice and development, Magnet project coordinator, Northwestern Memorial Hospital, Chicago

- Laura Caramanica, RN, PhD, vice president for nursing, Hartford Hospital, Hartford, CT

- Jody Childs, MBA, RN, nursing administrative specialist, Texas Children's Hospital, Houston

- Patricia Collins, RN, MSN, AOCN, Magnet coordinator, South Miami Hospital, Miami

- Cole Edmonson, MS, RN, CHE, CNAA, BC, associate administer of patient care services, Medical City Dallas Hospital and The North Texas Hospital for Children, Dallas

- Toni Fiore, MA, RN, CNAA, executive vice president, patient care and chief nursing officer, Hackensack University Medical Center, Hackensack, NJ

- Deborah Ford, RN, BSN, MSN, CNA, director of emergency services, Lafayette General Medical Center, Lafayette, LA

- Elaine Graf, RN, PhD, research and funding coordinator, clinical and organizational development, Children's Memorial Medical Center, Chicago

- Joanne Hambleton, RN, MSN, CNA, vice president of nursing and patient services, Fox Chase Cancer Center, Philadelphia

- Beverly Hancock, MS, RN, education/quality coordinator, Rush University Medical Center, Chicago

- Barbara Hannon, MSN, RN, Magnet coordinator, University of Iowa Hospitals and Clinics, Iowa City, IA

- Kim Hitchings, RN, MSN, manager, Center for Professional Excellence, clinical services, Lehigh Valley Hospital and Health Network, Allentown, PA

- Mary Ann Hozak, RN, BSN, CCRN, nurse manager SICU/OHRR, Saint Joseph's Regional Medical Center, Patterson, NJ

- Anne Jadwin, RN, MSN, AOCN, CNA, director of nursing, Fox Chase Cancer Center, Philadelphia

- Michelle Janney, RN, PhD, CNAA, chief nurse executive/vice president of operations, Northwestern Memorial Hospital, Chicago

- Janis Manis, RN, MS, Magnet coordinator, Miami Valley Hospital, Dayton, OH

- Susan H. Nick, RN, PhD, independent JCAHO/Magnet consultant, Chicago

- Sherill Nones Cronin, PhD, RN, BC, nurse researcher and Magnet coordinator, Jewish Hospital, Louisville, KY

- Susan Palette-Gallagher, MA, RN, CNAA, BC, administrative director of medical units and education, Community Medical Center, Toms River, NJ

- Diane Peyser, RN, MS, BC, CNA, Magnet project coordinator and director of staff development, Huntington Hospital, Huntington, NY

- Lisa Reiser, RN, MSN, chief nursing officer, University of California, Irvine Medical Center, Orange, CA

- Katherine Riley, BSN, RN, director, integrated clinical services, access services, women's and children's services, social services, and Magnet coordinator, Southwestern Vermont Medical Center, Bennington, VT

- Kim Sharkey, RN, MBA, CNAA, BC, Magnet site coordinator, Saint Joseph's Hospital of Atlanta, Atlanta

- Jane Shivnan, MScN, RN, AOCN, assistant director of nursing, oncology, The Sidney Kimmel Comprehensive Cancer Center at Johns Hopkins, Magnet project coordinator, The Johns Hopkins Hospital, Baltimore

- Barbara Smith, MSN, RN, BC, CNAA, BC, director of nursing, North Carolina Baptist Hospital of Wake Forest University Baptist Medical Center, Winston-Salem, NC

- Barbara Wadsworth, RN, MSN, CNAA, administrative nurse director, Abington Memorial Hospital, Abington, PA

- Kathryn "Ginger" Ward-Presson, RN, MSN, chief nurse executive/associate director of nursing, Miami VA Medical Center, Miami

- Elizabeth Warden, RN, CNA, MS, director of nursing, Forsyth Medical Center, Winston-Salem, NC

- Norine Watson, RN, MSN, corporate manager, service excellence, Christiana Care Health Services, Newark, DE

- Janet Wright, MSN, RN, BC, clinical nurse specialist, NorthEast Medical Center, Concord, NC

What is Magnet status and what are its benefits?

History of Magnet

During the nursing shortage of the 1980s, the American Academy of Nursing conducted a national research study to identify hospitals that had high retention rates and were able to recruit nurses despite the nursing shortage (McClure, Poulin, Sovie, & Wandelt, 2002). The study also attempted to identify organizational and nursing administration attributes that could be responsible for such success. As a result of this study, 41 "Magnet" hospitals were selected based on their ability to attract and retain registered nursing staff (McClure & Hinshaw, 2002).

These 41 Magnet hospitals shared the following organizational traits:

- The chief nurse executive (CNE) was a formal member of the highest decision-making body in the organization
- Nursing was organized as a relatively flat structure, with minimal layers of hierarchy
- Decision-making related to staffing and patient care was decentralized to include staff nurses at the unit level
- Administration supported the nurses' decisions regarding patient care
- Good communication existed between nurses and physicians (Havens & Aiken, 1999)

Research studies were conducted to provide empirical evidence that these hospitals had enhanced patient and nurse outcomes.

In the early 1990s, there was an emphasis on best practices, benchmarking, and quality outcomes data, as well as renewed interest in the Magnet concept. A need emerged to establish a process where healthcare organizations could apply for national recognition for excellence in nursing care.

Magnet's relationship to ANCC

In 1991, the American Nurses Credentialing Center (ANCC), a subsidiary of the American Nurses Association (ANA), was established to provide a process for both individuals and organizations to seek the accreditation, certification, and recognition the profession needed (Urden & Monarch, 2002). Thus, the ANCC established a process known as the Magnet Recognition Program™, to which hospitals could apply to be recognized as a center of nursing excellence.

The process consists of an initial application fee, submission of written documents exemplifying how the Forces of Magnetism—a list of quality indicators and standards of nursing practice—are incorporated into nursing services, participation in the National Database for Nursing Quality Indicators (NDNQI), and a multiday site visit. Additional expenses include appraisal fees, appraiser honorariums and travel fees, and site visit fees.

In 1994, the University of Washington Medical Center in Seattle became the first hospital to be awarded Magnet recognition by the ANCC. By 1998, 13 hospitals had been awarded Magnet recognition; only three were among the 41 identified in the 1980s (Havens & Aiken, 1999). As of August 2004, there were 105 Magnet designated hospitals—less than 2% of all hospitals in the country.

The growing interest in Magnet and the escalating rate of hospitals applying for it can be attributed to a number of factors:

1. Numerous published research studies have demonstrated better patient outcomes in hospitals with higher (i.e., better) nurse to patient ratios, higher percentages of certified nurses, and higher percentages of BSN-prepared nurses, all of which are characteristics of Magnet hospitals

2. Magnet has been identified in the federal Nurse Reinvestment Act and the Institute of Medicine Report as an initiative for reducing registered nurse turnover and improving quality of care

3. The Joint Commission on Accreditation of Healthcare Organizations (JCAHO) has identified Magnet as a positive force in improving practice environments, quality of care, and patient safety

4. Faculty in colleges and schools of nursing encourage graduates to ask questions regarding the practice environment of a potential employer and to seek employment at a Magnet hospital

5. In 2004, for the first time, Magnet was added as a factor in how U.S. News and World Report ranks hospitals

"Our standing in *U.S. News & World Report* as a comprehensive cancer center went up several notches this year due to our Magnet status. Believe me, we have tremendous buy-in here for the impact of nursing care on patient outcomes."

—Anne Jadwin, RN, MSN, AOCN, CNA

Perhaps most importantly, however, nurses want to be recognized for their excellent work, and Magnet provides that recognition. According to staff nurses, obtaining Magnet ensures that the voice of the nurse will be heard and appreciated.

Because the Magnet award only lasts for four years, organizations must recertify every four years to maintain Magnet status. The original Magnet Recognition Program has also expanded to include long-term care and international healthcare organizations. The ANCC's home page, *www.nursingworld.org,* includes the latest information and updates on the Magnet Recognition Program. To access it, click on the link for the ANCC and then click on Magnet Recognition.

Research related to Magnet

The original 41 hospitals were identified as Magnet facilities because of their ability to attract and retain registered nurses (RN). Descriptive research conducted in these hospitals produced a body of knowledge that defined the practice environments within them. These findings were presented in terms of attributes of the nursing leader, professional attributes of staff nurses, and the professional practice environment (Scott, Sochalski, & Aiken, 1999). Subsequent research studies validated and expanded these findings. They are summarized as follows (McClure & Hinshaw, 2002).

Nursing leaders

- are visionary and enthusiastic

- are supportive and knowledgeable

- maintain high practice standards

- value education and professional development

- hold positions of power and status within the organization

- are visible to staff nurses

- are actively involved in professional organizations

- respond to nurses' needs

- conduct open communication with staff nurses

Staff nurses

- have autonomy and are accountable for their practices

- can establish and maintain a positive nurse-patient relationship

- create collaborative nurse-physician relationships and conduct open communication

- participate in unit-based decision-making

- engage in patient teaching

- value the professional image of nursing

In a professional practice environment,

- the organization provides adequate staffing (from the perspective of the staff nurse)

- the nurse manager is supportive

- organizational support exists for education, professional growth, and career advancement

- nurses can participate in organizational decision-making

- nurses have competitive salaries and benefits

- nursing organization is decentralized

Due to their organizational support of nursing practices and their ability to attract and retain RNs, Magnet hospitals have higher (i.e., better) nurse-to-patient ratios. Key findings of major research studies that examine the relationship between nurse staffing and patient outcomes can be found in Figure 1.1.

| Figure 1.1 | Key findings of major research studies |

Author	Key findings
Aiken, et al.	• Magnet hospitals have decreased mortality rates, lengths of stay (LOS), and needle-stick injuries • Higher (better) nurse staffing was associated with lower mortality, fewer post-procedure complications, less failure to rescue, lower burnout rates, and higher nurse satisfaction • Higher proportion of nurses educated at baccalaureate level was associated with lower mortality and failure-to-rescue rates for surgical patients
Blegen, et al.	• Higher (better) nurse staffing was associated with decreased mortality, fewer medication errors, fewer patient falls, less skin breakdown, and increased patient satisfaction
ANA	• Higher (better) nurse staffing was associated with a decrease in LOS, pneumonia, urinary track infections, skin breakdown, and infections
Needleman, et al. (This study was instrumental in providing the definition of the nurse-sensitive indicators used for Magnet recognition)	• Higher (better) nurse staffing was associated with decreases in rate of failure to rescue, length of stay, pneumonia, GI bleed, shock, and cardiac arrest

Note: This is not meant to be an exhaustive reference list of research conducted in this area.

Benefits to nurses, patients, and the organization

Magnet is the highest level of recognition a hospital can achieve for excellence in nursing and is considered the "gold standard" in the nursing world. Although Magnet recognition is awarded for excellence exclusively in nursing services, its benefits extend to patients and to the organization as a whole. These benefits directly relate to the cultural transformation associated with obtaining and maintaining Magnet status and have been identified by research conducted in Magnet hospitals:

Benefits to nurses

- Autonomy in clinical practice decision-making
- Participation in nursing leadership and organizational decision-making
- Adequate nurse staffing
- Higher RN job satisfaction
- Enhanced nurse-physician collaboration
- Integration of professional models of care
- Decreased needle-stick injuries

Benefits to patients

- Decreased length of stay
- Increased patient/family satisfaction
- Decreased risk of falls, medication errors, postprocedure complications
- Confidence that the hospital has obtained the highest honor awarded for nursing care
- Reduced family complaints
- High quality of nursing care

Benefits to the organization

- Reduced RN turnover and vacancy rate
- Positive, collaborative, engaging work environment for all employees
- Competitive economic advantage—lower costs as a result of decreased RN turnover
- Ability to attract high-quality physicians (research documents that high-quality nursing is one of the most important attributes in attracting high-quality physicians)
- A culture built on empowerment, pride, mentoring, respect, integrity, caring, and teamwork, which emerges during the process
- Competitive marketing advantage
  - An article in the *Wall Street Journal* encouraged consumers to seek a Magnet hospital for treatment
  - ANCC encourages Magnet facilities to use this recognition as a way of marketing to consumers

References

Aiken, L. (2002). Superior outcomes for Magnet hospitals: The evidence base. In M. McClure & A. Hinshaw (Eds.), *Magnet hospitals revisited: Attraction and retention of registered nurses* (pp. 61–82). Washington, DC: American Nurses Publishing.

Aiken, L., Clarke, S., Cheung, R., Sloane, D., & Silber, J. (2003). Educational levels of hospital nurses and surgical patient mortality. *Journal of American Medical Association*, 209(12), 1617–1623.

Aiken, L., Clarke, S., Sloane, D., Sochalski, J., & Silber, J. (2002). Hospital nurse staffing and patient mortality, nurse burnout and job dissatisfaction. *Journal of American Medical Association*, 288(16), 1987–1993.

American Nurses Association (1997). *Implementing nursing's report card: A study of RN staffing, length of stay and patient outcomes*. Washington, DC: American Nurses Publishing.

American Nurses Association (2000). *Nurse staffing and patient outcomes in the inpatient hospital setting*. Report released by ANA.

Blegen, M., Goode, C., & Reed, L. (1998). Nurse staffing and patient outcomes. *Nursing Research*, 47(1), 43–50.

Blegen, M., & Vaughn, T. (1998). A multisite study of nurse staffing and patient outcomes. *Nursing Economics*, 16(4), 196–203.

Havens, D., & Aiken, L. (1999). Shaping systems to promote desired outcomes: The Magnet hospital model. *Journal of Nursing Administration*, 29(2), 14–20.

McClure, M., & Hinshaw, A. (Eds.) (2002). *Magnet hospitals revisited: Attraction and retention of professional nurses*. Washington, DC: American Nurses Publishing.

McClure, M., Poulin, A., Sovie, M., & Wandelt, M. (2002). Magnet hospitals: Attraction and retention of professional nurses (the original study). In M. McClure & A. Hinshaw (Eds.), *Magnet hospitals revisited: Attraction and retention of professional nurses* (pp. 1–24). Washington, DC: American Nurses Publishing.

Needleman, J., Buerhaus, P., Mattke, S., Stewart, M., & Zelevinsky, K. (2002). Nurse staffing levels and the quality of care in hospitals. *The New England Journal of Medicine, 346*(22), 1715–1722.

Scott, J., Sochalski, J., & Aiken, L. (1999). Review of Magnet hospital research: Findings and implications for professional nursing practice. *Journal of Nursing Administration, 29*(1), 9–19.

Urden, L., & Monarch, K. (2002). The ANCC Magnet recognition program: Converting research findings into action. In M. McClure & A. Hinshaw (Eds.), *Magnet hospitals revisited: Attraction and retention of professional nurses* (pp. 103–15). Washington, DC: American Nurses Publishing.

Assessing and communicating Magnet status within your organization

Key points to consider before a decision is made

It is important to note that once you submit the $2,500 nonrefundable application fee and one-page application to the Magnet Program Office, your organization has two years to complete and submit the written documents. To ensure compliance with this deadline, your chief nurse executive (CNE) must assess whether the organization is ready to apply or needs to spend one to two years in a pre-planning phase, implementing needed cultural transformation and identifying processes by which to collect required data.

For organizations with processes in place that exemplify the 14 Forces of Magnetism, the Magnet journey and final recognition will reflect the nursing excellence already in place. Organizations that need to make changes and set up processes, however, can use the 14 Forces of Magnetism as a framework for such change and to guide nursing practice.

Once the CNE has expressed an interest in pursuing Magnet designation, he or she should purchase a manual and review the standards. This will help him or her determine the level of organizational readiness.

The assessment tool in Figure 2.1 is based on some of the 14 Forces of Magnetism and practice exemplars that will be evaluated during either document review or the site visit. Please note that this tool is meant to be an initial assessment of organizational readiness. It does not replace the detailed gap analysis, which we will discuss in Chapter 5.

Figure 2.1

Magnet readiness assessment tool

Question	Yes	No
Is the position of chief nurse officer (CNO) at the executive level of the organization?		
Do the *Scope and Standards for Nurse Administrators* (ANA, 2003) serve as a framework for practice?		
Is the nursing organizational structure generally flat, with staff nurses involved in unit-based decision-making?		
Do staff nurses actively participate in decision-making committees at the organizational level?		
Are nursing leaders actively involved in professional organizations?		
Does evidence-based practice guide nursing policies/procedures and clinical decision-making?		
Are there committees at the nursing level (e.g., nursing practice council, nursing education council) composed of staff nurses where practice decisions are made?		
Does the organization collect data at the unit level on nursing-sensitive indicators (e.g., nurse satisfaction, falls, pressure ulcers, patient satisfaction, skill-mix, and nursing care hours/patient day)?		
Are you willing to participate in a national database, which requires collection and submission of the above? (Required)		
Is there a mechanism(s) in place to support registered nurses in obtaining professional certification?		
Does the organization provide opportunities for the professional growth and development of staff nurses?		
Does the CNO have a master's degree? (Required) (Effective February 2008, the CNO's either baccalaureate or master's degree must be in nursing)		
Are staff nurses actively involved in professional organizations?		
Is there an active nursing research council in place?		
Do the majority of staff nurses feel they have adequate staff to provide quality patient care?		
In the five years preceding the application, has the organization committed an unfair labor practice? (If yes, please contact the ANCC to discuss eligibility) (Required)		

There is no magical, correct number of responses to the questions in Figure 2.1; however, all organizations must answer appropriately on the required items. If you have answered "yes" to the majority of the questions, the organization will be able to move forward more quickly in the process. If you answered "no" to the majority of the questions, give yourself at least two years to implement strategic goals to meet these criteria and work on cultural transformation. It is important to give yourself the time you need to create a culture of nursing excellence that reflects the Forces of Magnetism.

Don't get discouraged at this point. Instead, use the assessment process as an opportunity to enhance the practice environment. The amount of time it takes to make these changes depends on many contextual issues within the organization and varies between organizations. For example, if you don't have a nursing research council in place, consider the following as you move forward in the process:

- Does the organization have a master's or doctoral-prepared RN to lead the council?
- Does the library have a variety of scholarly and professional nursing journals?
- Are members of the nursing staff able to access electronic journals from the nursing units?
- Does the organization have consultants available to guide the council? Is there a charge for these services?
- Are faculty from a local college or university willing to serve as mentors to the nursing staff for research initiatives?
- Will the hospital institutional review board (IRB) provide support and guidance to the nursing research council?

The availability of resources will vary, but the more internal and external resources available, the more quickly the CNE can move the process forward.

"The Magnet initiative was a vision of the vice president, operations/chief nurse executive. A diverse committee of 25 was led by co-chairs. The committee conducted an assessment of the organization, reviewed the standards, prepared the application, communicated to all hospital disciplines, and prepared everyone for the site visit."

—Barbara Smith, MSN, RN, BC, CNAA, BC

Key points for engaging the leadership team

To achieve a successful Magnet journey, the hospital's CNE must gain support and commitment from the leadership team. Although Magnet recognizes excellence in nursing services, the nursing practice environment does not exist in a vacuum, apart from the rest of the organization. Hold a strategic planning meeting during the preplanning phase with members of the leadership team to discuss the cultural transformation and what specific tasks need to be accomplished to obtain and sustain Magnet status.

Most CNEs have found it helpful to do a high-level presentation early in the process to educate, excite, and engage the team. They then do a second, more detailed presentation as a follow-up, to discuss the specific involvement of the various leaders and departments to ensure organizational success. Examples of concepts to be included in both the initial and follow-up presentations are listed below.

Topics to include in initial presentation
- History and background of Magnet recognition
- Identification of hospitals in your market that have achieved Magnet status
- Relationship of Magnet to other regulatory agencies/federal reports
- Relevance of obtaining Magnet status to your organization
- Interrelationship between Forces of Magnetism and your organizational initiatives
- Benefits to patients, employees, and the organization
- Costs and economic benefits associated with Magnet
- How your organization compares to Magnet organizations (in terms of RN turnover, RN vacancy, patient outcome data, etc.)
- Brief overview of needed cultural transformation

Topics for follow-up presentation
- Support required from
  - data management (quality department)
  - informatics infrastructure (IT department)
  - RN demographic data (human resource [HR] department)

- willingness to accept cultural changes (i.e., active involvement of staff nurses in hospital committees/organizational decision-making)
- public relations/marketing department

• Overview of the phases of the Magnet recognition process

• Committee structure and responsibilities

• Organizational events (e.g., kick-off event, Magnet fairs, etc.)

• Interdisciplinary collaboration

• Final budget for three years

• Economic investment in the future

"To get a buy-in, you must tie the group you are speaking to into the overall goal by letting them see how Magnet designation will help them. For example, I made a PowerPoint presentation on 'nurse-physician collegiality' that was built around the acute nursing shortage, which certainly affects physicians at the hospital. I emphasized how important it was to retain each and every nurse at the hospital and how physicians could help create a more collegial environment that might ensure nurses not leaving because of physician issues. This PowerPoint was taken to every clinical faculty group at the hospital and was well-received, with most faculty groups expressing a desire to make the environment more nurse-physician friendly. I also talked to groups like 'dietary,' asking for their support. Letting dietary be a part of the Magnet effort was important and letting them know we could not get Magnet recognition without their services made them feel included in the all the excitement. Include everyone, do not make this only a nursing initiative, after all, nursing does not practice in a vacuum."

—Barbara Hannon, MSN, RN

"In order to achieve buy-in, you should attend medical board, executive board, and department-head meetings. Use the chief executive officer (CEO) and chief medical officer (CMO) to gain support for the project. It is indeed a hospital award, not a nursing award, and we continued to emphasize that point."

—Mary Ann Hozak, RN, BSN, CCRN

Cost-benefit assessment

Organizational costs will vary by organization. CNEs will need to decide either to use internal resources or to depend on external resources. If they decide to rely on internal resources, they must realize that the time and energy devoted to Magnet may mean other initiatives don't get priority or nursing leaders have to assist in cross-covering areas of responsibility. Figure 2.2 can serve as a guide to determine costs within your organization.

Figure 2.2

Fixed costs related to Magnet recognition (based on an organization with 400–499 beds)

Initial application fee	$2,500.00
Site-visit appraisal fee (cost depends on size of organization)	$30,450.00
Appraiser honorarium (based on two appraisers at $1,000 per appraiser; large organizations may require additional appraisers)	$2,000.00
Site-visit fee (based on two appraisers for two full days at $1,500 per day per appraiser; large organizations or organizations with multiple sites may require more days)	$6,000.00
Travel expenses for appraisers for site visit (based on two appraisers at $1,500 per appraiser; includes airfare, lodging, food, transportation)	$3,000.00
Participation in National Database of Nursing Quality Indicators (NDNQI) database (for two full years of participation)	$7,000.00
Total	**$50,950.00**
The cost to recruit one nurse can be up to $60,000	

The fixed costs may increase slightly over the next few years, so check the application manual or ANCC Web site for the exact costs when your organization is ready to apply. The initial nonrefundable application fee of $2,500 is due when the organization decides to apply. The site-visit appraisal fee is due when the written documents are submitted. Applicants will be invoiced for the appraiser honorarium when the documents are being reviewed and the site-visit fee will be invoiced once the site-visit dates have been identified.

Applicants for Magnet must collect data on nurse-sensitive quality indicators, and these data must be submitted to a national database for benchmarking purposes. The center currently collecting this data is the National Database for Nursing Quality Indicators (NDNQI). Participants must collect and submit two sets of data for the appraisers to review. This process usually occurs over two full years. However, if an organization submits data in the second, third, or fourth quarter, there is a slight fee reduction for the first year. Participation for a second year requires the fee for the entire year.

All members of the leadership team must support the financial budget necessary to obtain Magnet. For this to occur, leaders must see the larger perspective and the importance of Magnet—the recognition should not be valued only by nursing. Some organizations have received the initial funds to finance Magnet from grants, their foundations, or private donors. Others have used funds from the operations budget to cover the expenses. The table in Figure 2.3 shows the optional costs related to Magnet recognition.

Figure 2.3 | **Optional costs related to Magnet**

Attending national workshop and research conference (four participants at $2,000 per participant)	$8,000.00
Attending regional workshops (four participants at $500 per participant)	$2,000.00
Brochures, posters, and promotional materials	$5,000.00
Organizational events (cost for light snacks and giveaways)	$5,000.00
Honorarium for external reviewer to read and edit final document	$2,000.00
Magnet Project Coordinator (1.0 FTE) ($80,000 per year for two years)*	$160,000.00
Staff nurse committee involvement can range from $0–$115,200 per year*	$230,400.00
Secretarial support (0.5 FTE: document preparation, preparing for site-visit; $25,000 per year with partial benefits)	$50,000.00
Consultative fees (assist with gap analysis, review of final documents, $13,000 per year for two years)	$26,000.00
Total	**$488,400.00**

*Denotes detailed discussion in narrative

The CNE must evaluate the optional costs to determine what will work best for the organization. For example, many feel that it has been extremely important to send the Magnet Project Coordinator, a member of the nursing leadership team, and two staff nurses to the Annual Magnet Conference co-sponsored by the ANCC. This is a wonderful opportunity to hear how other Magnet organizations have prepared for their "journey to excellence" and to network with nursing leaders and staff nurses from other Magnet facilities.

Prior to this national conference, the ANCC, in conjunction with Institute for Research, Education, and Consultation (IREC), hosts a Magnet workshop at which organizations interested in applying for Magnet can learn how to both interpret the Forces of Magnetism and prepare for application and site visit. In addition to the workshop preceding the conference, there are local two-day workshops hosted by the ANCC in most major cities at various times during the year. Staff nurses who have attended these workshops have a better understanding of the challenges, rewards, and specific activities associated with Magnet.

Other optional expenses include brochures, posters, promotional materials, and organizational events, which promote organizational awareness of what is involved in achieving Magnet and engage all employees in the process. Some organizations host a major kickoff event to obtain volunteers, some host events during the process to showcase progress, and others have a Magnet fair before the site visit. Brochures and posters communicate the organization's progress to employees and the community. Promotional materials such as pens, cups, or calendars can include the organization's unique theme or saying related to Magnet. They can be given to new employees, used at recruitment fairs, or be awarded as prizes for individuals or units making unique contributions to the Magnet journey.

The major optional costs include those associated with a dedicated Magnet Project Coordinator, time for staff nurses to be involved in committees and Magnet planning, and secretarial support related to document preparation. In making these decisions, the CNE needs to consider the availability of human and economic resources. The following lists serve as guides through the decision-making process.

Magnet Project Coordinator

A dedicated full-time equivalent (FTE) can

- be committed to Magnet 100% and able to honor timelines
- create consistency—one writer, one voice
- guide the process and chair the steering committee
- oversee data collection of nurse-sensitive indicators
- establish a process by which to collect registered nurse demographics
- be an ad hoc member of Magnet committees

Alternatives to a dedicated FTE that have been used in Magnet facilities include the following:

- A member of the nursing leadership team serves in this role. Other members of the team assist with his or her operational duties. Cost is budget-neutral and remains in the nursing operation budget.
- A steering committee accepts responsibility for many of the tasks, so members spend only 25% of their effort on the project as part of their professional responsibilities. Cost is budget-neutral.
- Members of the nursing leadership team divide tasks and writing as part of their professional responsibility. The project is a collaborative effort. Cost remains budget-neutral. In this case, an external reader must review and edit all documents so they are in one voice and one writing style.
- Nursing director or nurse manager assumes the role of Magnet Project Coordinator at 100% effort. They are replaced for the next two years by an internal candidate serving in the role on an interim basis. The cost of a leader assuming the role of Magnet Project Coordinator is charged to the Magnet budget; the replacement cost remains in the nursing operation budget.

Costs for staff nurse participation

Determining the costs of staff nurse participation in nursing committees and assistance with Magnet varies immensely among organizations. In organizations focused on career ladders and professional development, participation is expected in professional practice, and staff are not compensated for committee participation. In other organizations, eight hours of professional development per nurse has been built into the operational budget, and during the Magnet journey, this time is devoted to active involvement and participation in Magnet projects and committees. At times, creativity is needed to remain budget-neutral. In one Magnet facility, the nursing leadership team and unit managers assisted with unit coverage to allow staff nurses to attend meetings and work on Magnet projects.

The size and complexity of the organization is a major consideration when planning the costs associated with active participation of staff nurses. A small hospital (i.e., less than 200 beds) may need fewer committees to accomplish Magnet projects, whereas larger organizations may need more committees and staff nurse participation to ensure representation from all areas of the organization.

The CNE also must consider how to restructure the meeting times of hospital-wide committees to allow for staff nurse participation. For example, in one organization, the ethics committee always met at 7:30 a.m., which made it difficult for a staff RN to attend. Changing the time to 8 a.m. allowed for an emergency room night shift RN to become an active participant of this committee.

For illustration purposes, the figure of $115,200 (total annual cost for staff nurse committee involvement) was calculated as follows: five practice councils x eight staff/council x 48 hours/year (four hours/month) = 1,920 hours x $30/hour replacement costs = $57,600. For participation in Magnet committee/projects, the same formula is used: five Magnet committees x eight staff/committee x 48 hours/year = 1,920 hours x $30/hour replacement costs = $57,600, or $115,200/year.

This figure is not meant to be an absolute, but it is rather an initial dollar amount for discussion and review. Some CNEs have stated that the allocated hours for staff nurse participation on committees and on Magnet projects was equal to two times a manager's salary for a year in their organization. Our figure provides an estimate of associated costs, with a rationale based on the number of hours staff nurses have contributed in other Magnet facilities. It is also based on organizations that have no active staff nurse-driven committees in place. Those that have active staff nurse committees in place are ready to take on additional responsibilities related to Magnet.

For example, one organization that has just started its Magnet journey had an education council in place. Their primary responsibility was to review nursing orientation practices and recommend classes for continuing education at the hospital. They always met once a month at lunch time and communicated via hospital e-mail in the interim. The committee was always budget-neutral. When the announcement was made concerning Magnet, the chair approached the CNE and said the committee would take on additional responsibilities to focus on educating the nurses on Magnet. As a group, they decided that they could do their orientation and CEU review via hospital e-mail. They also realized the need to have increased night-shift involvement and set out to increase off-shift participation.

Secretarial support

Some organizations decide to hire temporary, external secretarial support. Even those that don't, however, must know that preparing the documents for review by the appraisers and gathering the documents needed for the site visit is labor-intensive. Once the organization is actively involved in the Magnet process, it will probably need external support or, to remain budget-neutral, it can assign a secretary already in place to assist with Magnet.

The amount of work varies from 10 to 40 hours a week, depending on the scope and depth of the documents. Some larger organizations, or those going up as a system, have designated secretarial support on a full-time basis. In any case, maintain consistency in the process; that is, employ one designated secretary instead of sharing the workload on a rotational basis. The secretary working on Magnet projects should be extremely proficient in Microsoft Word, Excel, PowerPoint, and formatting large data sets.

External consultants

Many organizations find it valuable to have an external consultant assist with the gap analysis and timeline to complete projects. Another way to use a consultant is to review the final documents for adherence to the Forces of Magnetism, consistency in style, and logical flow. The consultant needs to be familiar with the Forces of Magnetism to verify that the exemplars submitted reflect the best nursing practices of the organization and meet the application manual's criteria.

Return on investment considerations

Magnet can be expensive, especially in terms of the human and economic resources necessary to transform the culture and enhance the practice environment, but facilities can't afford not to do it.

Key benefits:

- Cost to recruit and replace one nurse ($60,000) (Advisory Board Company)
- Decreased RN turnover rate and vacancy rate
- Eliminated or decreased use of agency nurses
- Decreased adverse events (associated with high-cost interventions)
- Increased community recognition in terms of endowments
- Better preparation for JCAHO requirements in terms of nursing documentation
- Magnet status considered in terms of bond rating and risk management assessment

Staff nurse practice environment

A major characteristic of Magnet hospitals is the ability of the nursing leadership team to create an environment that empowers and respects nursing staff. The accreditation process ensures that Magnet facilities live up to this standard.

A large portion of the submitted documentation and site-visit appraisal needs to reflect the role of the staff nurse. As part of the organizational assessment, you might find it useful to see what grade you made on all or some of the questions found in Figure 2.4.

All members of the nursing leadership team should take this assessment first. The second phase includes a random distribution to 10% of the RNs providing direct patient care. The items come from research on staff nurses conducted by Kramer and Schmalenberg (2002). The concept of assigning a grade to the score was developed by the author and reviewed by CNEs who have achieved Magnet.

Figure 2.4	Making the grade: Essentials of Magnetism

Instructions: For each question, please rate the hospital in which you currently practice. For members of the leadership team, consider what staff nurses providing direct care would say. A score of 10 is 100%, or perfect, while a score of 1 is 10%, or absolute failure/terrible.

1. Working with other nurses who are clinically competent.

Terrible   Perfect

☐   ☐   ☐   ☐   ☐   ☐   ☐   ☐   ☐   ☐

1   2   3   4   5   6   7   8   9   10

2. Good nurse-physician relationships and communication.

Terrible   Perfect

☐   ☐   ☐   ☐   ☐   ☐   ☐   ☐   ☐   ☐

1   2   3   4   5   6   7   8   9   10

3. Nurse autonomy and accountability.

Terrible   Perfect

☐   ☐   ☐   ☐   ☐   ☐   ☐   ☐   ☐   ☐

1   2   3   4   5   6   7   8   9   10

| Figure 2.4 | Making the grade: Essentials of Magnetism (cont.) |

4. Supportive nurse manager.

Terrible   Perfect

☐   ☐   ☐   ☐   ☐   ☐   ☐   ☐   ☐   ☐
1   2   3   4   5   6   7   8   9   10

5. Control over nursing practices and practice environment.

Terrible   Perfect

☐   ☐   ☐   ☐   ☐   ☐   ☐   ☐   ☐   ☐
1   2   3   4   5   6   7   8   9   10

6. Support for education (in-service, continuing education, tuition, etc.).

Terrible   Perfect

☐   ☐   ☐   ☐   ☐   ☐   ☐   ☐   ☐   ☐
1   2   3   4   5   6   7   8   9   10

7. Adequate nurse staffing.

Terrible   Perfect

☐   ☐   ☐   ☐   ☐   ☐   ☐   ☐   ☐   ☐
1   2   3   4   5   6   7   8   9   10

8. Concern for the patient is paramount.

Terrible   Perfect

☐   ☐   ☐   ☐   ☐   ☐   ☐   ☐   ☐   ☐
1   2   3   4   5   6   7   8   9   10

9. Visibility of chief nurse executive.

Terrible   Perfect

☐   ☐   ☐   ☐   ☐   ☐   ☐   ☐   ☐   ☐
1   2   3   4   5   6   7   8   9   10

10. Staff nurse participation in hospital committees.

Terrible   Perfect

☐   ☐   ☐   ☐   ☐   ☐   ☐   ☐   ☐   ☐
1   2   3   4   5   6   7   8   9   10

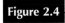

Figure 2.4 | **Making the grade: Essentials of Magnetism (cont.)**

Interpretation of results: Your score (individual questions)

100%	Perfect A+	Identify practice exemplars to support, ready to write on this criterion
90%	A	Identify practice exemplars to support, ready to write on this criterion
80%	B	Moving forward, work on weaknesses and then start writing on this criterion
70%	C	Potential is there, minor to moderate cultural transformation needed
Below 70%		Major cultural transformation needed

Overall score

100%	Perfect A+	Ready to apply.
90%	A	In great shape, ready to apply.
80%	B	In good shape, ready to apply. Evaluate weakness, seek staff nurse input to enhance.
70%–60%	C	Work on cultural transformation, seek staff nurse input. Reevaluate staff in six months. If improvement noted, ready to apply.
Below 60%		Major cultural transformation required. Work on changes for 12–24 months before applying.

Certification

Part of the requested demographics for Magnet is identification of the number of RNs who have achieved national certification. This information is required for each individual unit and distinguishes among RNs providing direct patient care, RNs not providing direct patient care, and advanced practice nurses.

In Magnet hospitals, 26.4% of all direct care RNs are certified in at least one specialty (Monarch, 2003). Before applying for Magnet, determine the number of certified direct care RNs within your facility. Certification is defined as being designated by a nationally or internationally recognized certifying organization. For this purpose, cardiopulmonary resuscitation (CPR), advanced cardiac life support (ACLS), and pediatric advanced life support (PALS) are considered technical certifications and are not counted in the certification database. Strategies for increasing the number of nurses certified within your organization include

- using tuition reimbursement funds to cover the external review course and the cost of the examination
- compensating for time off-unit to attend the review course or take the exam
- holding review courses free of charge at the hospital
- purchasing study guides or textbooks for reference
- clinical ladder advancement
- recognition during nurses' week
- salary increase
- recognition on performance appraisal
- paying for staff to attend off-site review courses

References

Advisory Board Company, Nurse Executive Center (2002). *Reversing the flight of talent: Nursing retention in an era of gathering shortages*. Washington, DC.

Kramer, M., & Schmalenberg, C. (2002). Staff nurses identify essentials of magnetism. In M. McClure & A. Hinshaw (Eds.). *Magnet hospitals revisited: Attraction and retention of professional nurses* (pp. 25–59). Washington, DC: American Nurses Publishing.

Monarch, K. (2003). Magnet hospitals: Powerful force for excellence. *Reflections on nursing leadership*. Fourth quarter, 10–13.

Preparing for the process

Your timeline

Once you have identified organizational readiness based on the self-assessment and staff nurse practice environment assessment (see Figure 2.4 in Chapter 2), set up a realistic timeline.

Remember, once the initial one-page application and $2,500 fee is sent in, you have two years (24 months) to submit the completed application. If, based on your assessment, your organization is not ready to apply for Magnet, a cultural transformation must occur, and that alone can take up to 24 months. Therefore, be sure your organization is culturally prepared ahead of time. Develop the timeline with input from key contributors to the process within your organization. The timeline needs to be realistic and reflect consensus to avoid making members of the team feel stressed or overburdened with the prospect of adhering to it. Remember, the Magnet process is an experience and a journey, not a race to see how quickly your organization can complete the documents.

Once the initial application is sent in, the clock starts, and the organization has two years to send in all supporting documents. Although the journey is exciting and rewarding, it can also become difficult, labor-intensive, and tedious. Therefore, set the date for the final submission of documents 18–20 months after the initial application. Doing so allows for ongoing reassessment and dialogue among the Magnet team to evaluate progress and to make necessary changes that have been identified by the outside reviewer or consultant. If difficulties or unexplained issues arise, it leaves you time to deal with them without creating additional stress or tension to meet the deadline.

Figure 3.1 is a timeline from Rush University Medical Center in Chicago, which was awarded Magnet recognition on May 31, 2002.

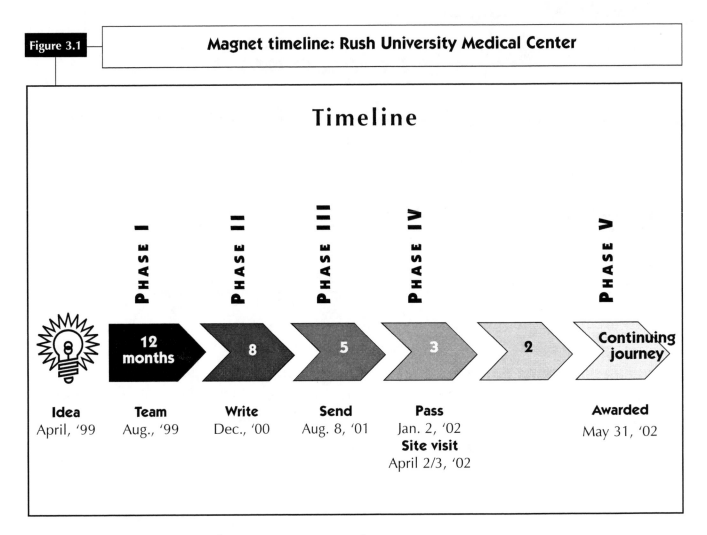

Figure 3.1 — **Magnet timeline: Rush University Medical Center**

Timeline

PHASE I — 12 months — Idea April, '99 / Team Aug., '99

PHASE II — 8 — Write Dec., '00

PHASE III — 5 — Send Aug. 8, '01

PHASE IV — 3 — Pass Jan. 2, '02 / Site visit April 2/3, '02

2

PHASE V — Continuing journey — Awarded May 31, '02

Committee structure (nurse autonomy)

Based on the literature and practice environments focused on shared governance and a decentralized management model, the following committee structure can be used as a model for committees that should be in place and functioning for at least one year prior to applying for Magnet. In addition to participating in nursing committees, staff nurses need to be active members of interdisciplinary hospital committees.

Having these committees in place will make it easy to identify practice exemplars that reflect of the Forces of Magnetism, especially autonomy and professional models of care. The documentation submitted for Magnet status reflects the work and outcomes of these committees or councils. Without a solid framework in place, however, your organization will not be able to move forward in the process.

Whether to identify these structures as committees or councils is an individual organizational decision. However, staff nurses often feel more empowered when the term "council" is used. They feel they are making decisions rather than just attending a committee meeting. The specific names, numbers, and exact responsibilities of each committee will vary by organization, depending on its size and the availability of resources.

Key committees or councils

Nursing practice council (nursing quality council)
- is responsible for evidence-based policies and procedures
- reviews new products for use in patient-care areas
- processes requests for changes in practice
- reviews sentinel events and adverse events to initiate change in practice
- assists with regulatory compliance (JCAHO)
- oversees unit-based quality projects

Nursing education council
- reviews new employee orientation
- suggests/evaluates continuing education offerings
- reviews required competencies and develops implementation plan for annual competency evaluation
- identifies strategies to increase certification and professional development
- assists in development of patient/family education material

Nursing research council
- writes guidelines for establishing journal clubs
- develops guidelines for critique of journal articles
- prepares criteria for submission of research proposals
- reviews and approves all nursing research studies prior to submission to hospital institutional review board (IRB)
- incorporates research findings into practice
- organizes internal research conference
- develops research-focused criteria for performance appraisal

Nursing recruitment and retention council (also known as nursing recognition council or nursing practice environment council)

- reviews/revises staffing, scheduling, and floating policies
- provides input to human resources (HR) on nursing compensation and benefits
- organizes retention initiatives
- attends recruitment job fairs
- plans nursing recognition events

Nursing leadership council

- participates in the formulation of the budget for nursing resources
- participates in strategic planning for nursing
- reviews/revises nursing philosophy as needed
- contributes to the process for clinical ladders and peer/self evaluations
- reviews patient and nurse satisfaction surveys and recommends practice changes

Magnet committees or task forces

You may decide to reassign the workload to existing committees or to set up new committees (task forces) related to Magnet. Some organizations do the latter in order to increase staff nurse involvement in the process and to allow the committees already in place to move forward with their original goals and objectives.

Other organizations may have committees that have existed for a while and are looking for new challenges. If this is the case, simply adding staff nurses and other members of the interdisciplinary team to the existing committees may be sufficient to accomplish the projects that are part of the Magnet journey.

Create a Magnet steering committee that meets quarterly in the year prior to the application process and then monthly for full-day meetings while the documentation is being compiled. During meetings, familiarize staff with evidence-based Magnet literature, the Forces of Magnetism, and the standards necessary to maintain the recognition. Encourage staff to compile evidence of compliance.

To ensure efficiency and effective time management at the meetings, break your staff into work groups and have them address sections of the standards in detail. They should be responsible for generating evidence of compliance with the standards and for documenting the sources clearly. Include in your committee CNSs, nurse researchers, managers, and staff nurses from every area in which nursing care is delivered. "We wanted extensive staff involvement so that the department was fully represented, informed, and involved."

—Anne Jadwin, RN, MSN, AOCN, CNA

Below is an example of the Magnet committee structure developed by Janet Cahill, RN, BSN, MBA, director of professional practice and development and Magnet project coordinator for Northwestern Memorial Hospital in Chicago. Cahill devised the concept of having committee chairs and organizing the committees under the major headings of

- quality
- Forces of Magnetism
- marketing/education

Subcommittees have been identified under each major heading and have a team leader to serve as facilitator. The committee chairs are vice presidents within the organization, so they serve as resources and guides for the team leaders. They are also members of the steering committee.

Northwestern Memorial Hospital is a large academic medical center (over 700 beds), so this structure provides a mechanism by which the steering committee receives information from the individual committees, but each team leader is not a member of the steering committee.

The sample committee structure in Figure 3.2 covers all of the related tasks or projects needed for both document and site-visit preparation. Cahill views the overall committee structure as a puzzle. "Each committee is a piece of the puzzle, and when all the pieces of the puzzle come together, our work, i.e., successful document and site-visit review, is complete. We now have a picture of nursing excellence unique to Northwestern Memorial Hospital."

Figure 3.2	Sample committee structure

Steering committee

Quality	Forces	Marketing and education
Organizational overview	Organizational structure and management style	Nursing education and integration
NDNQI	Quality of care and improvement	Marketing and PR
Nurse-sensitive indicators	Professional models of care and autonomy	Community
	Nurse as a teacher and community and the hospital	
	Professional image of nursing and personal policies	
	Interdisciplinary relationships and consultation and resources	
	Quality of leadership and professional development	

The steering committee membership at Northwestern Memorial Hospital includes

- chief nurse executive (1)
- committee chairs (4)
- senior vice president for human resources (1)
- Magnet project coordinator (1)
- Magnet project consultant (1)
- staff nurses (i.e., direct care givers) (2)
- advanced practice nurse (APN) (1)
- member of the medical staff (1)

Although Magnet recognizes excellence in nursing, Michelle Janney, RN, PhD, chief nurse executive and vice president of operations at Northwestern Memorial Hospital, expanded the framework to include "excellence in patient care and the organization as a whole." Her vision from the beginning was to enhance interdisciplinary support, participation, and involvement in the Magnet journey. To accomplish this vision, Janney presented her strategic plan to the senior leadership team and then invited nonnursing vice presidents to serve as committee chairs and steering committee members. The vice president of quality is the committee chair for quality; the senior vice president for women's health and vice president of operations are the committee chairs for the Forces of Magnetism committee; and the vice president of public relations, marketing, and physician services is the committee chair for marketing/education. All welcomed the opportunity to showcase the organization. Members of other disciplines and physicians serve as team leaders or active committee members.

Making this an organizational journey rather than a nursing journey has proven successful at Northwestern. Vice presidents and members of the senior leadership team not serving on committees volunteer to help as needed and encourage their departments to assist in the process. For example, the finance department is more than willing to provide organizational data on case-mix index and average daily census. The quality and risk management departments are involved in collecting the required quality and nurse-sensitive indicators and representatives from these departments serve as members of the committee responsible for these projects. According to Janney, "We are already seeing the engagement and excitement throughout the organization and will keep this focus throughout our journey."

This example serves as a reference and can be modified to reflect the needs of your organization. At minimum, organizations should consider having at least four committees to accomplish the needed tasks associated with Magnet. These include a

1. quality committee
2. Forces of Magnetism committee
3. education/marketing committee
4. steering committee

One of the best things Christiana Care Health Services did was form a Magnet executive team. Vice presidents gathered together monthly to discuss how they could support the nursing team in its pursuit of this recognition. The executive team was involved every step of the way—and even celebrated when the documentation had been submitted. Forming this team was particularly helpful because anyone working for the various vice presidents understands the Magnet process and readily complies with any requests made by those pursuing Magnet status.

—Norine Watson, RN, MSN

Determining committee membership

The following is a list of guiding principles that are important when determining committee membership:

- Committees need to be interdisciplinary
- The ideal committee size is eight to 12 members
- The majority of members should be registered nurses (RNs) who provide direct patient care
- Ensure a balance between detailed planners and creative thinkers
- Staff nurses can serve as committee chairs or share the role with a member of the nursing leadership team
- Patient-care technicians, nursing assistants, unit clerks, and licensed practical nurses are valuable contributors, so remember to include them
- Members of the nursing leadership team and the Magnet project coordinator should serve as resources and ad hoc committee members

Committee expectations

Once committee membership has been decided, have either the Magnet project coordinator or chair of the steering committee meet with the chairs to review committee expectations and responsibilities. Doing so is essential to ensure continuity, goal accomplishment, and adherence to the timeline.

Members often want to know how frequently the committee will meet before they agree to serve as members. There is no hard and fast rule for this, but in the beginning, committees should meet at least once or twice a month. The committee chair will need to reevaluate progress on a regular basis and determine whether the committee is meeting the established deadlines for project completion.

Committee expectations include

- commitment to honoring timeline
- full engagement and participation of all members during the meeting
- respectful, open communication style
- commitment from members to attend meetings
- set time for future meetings at first meeting
- rotate role of secretary unless one member enjoys taking minutes

Committee responsibilities

The following list provides some high-level committee responsibilities and is not meant to be an exhaustive list of projects for which the committee is responsible.

This list is based on having the minimum number of four committees, focusing on quality, Forces of Magnetism, marketing/education, and a steering committee. You can expand or decrease the number of committees or refocus the responsibilities based on your organization's preference.

Often, the quality committee is referred to as "the detailed committee" because of the enormous amount of specific information they are responsible for collecting and submitting. The Forces of Magnetism committee is viewed as "the writing committee," and the marketing/education committee is known as the "fun committee." The steering committee is known as the "overview" or "leadership" committee.

Quality committee

- Collects and submits required data for participation in National Database of Nursing Quality Indicators (NDNQI)
- Collects and submits unit-level, nurse-sensitive indicators
- Establishes process for distribution of nurse-satisfaction survey
- Participates in collection of organizational demographic data
- Participates in collection of unit-based RN demographic data
- Disseminates results of NDNQI participation and recommends practice changes

Forces of Magnetism committee(s)

There are 14 Forces, and the number of committees working to achieve them varies among organizations. For example, some organizations have one committee, while others have as many as seven, with each committee responsible for two of the forces. The committees

- provide practice examples and collect supporting evidence from the point of care on how the Forces are integrated across nursing services.
- draft written documentation for submission to the steering committee/Magnet project coordinator.

Marketing/education committee

- Identifies organization theme
- Develops brochures, posters, and flyers to keep employees aware of the project's progress
- Writes Magnet update articles for employee and nursing newsletters
- Educates all members of the organization on Magnet
- Identifies unit-based "cheerleaders," "champions," or "ambassadors" to keep the nursing staff energized
- Channels concerns of nursing staff to steering committee
- Prepares organization for site visit
- Coordinates organizational events or Magnet fairs
- Develops internal Web site highlighting how Forces of Magnetism are practiced across nursing services

Steering committee

- Assists chief nurse executive in evaluating organizational readiness
- Leads application process including document submission and site visit
- Conducts brainstorming sessions for members of all the Magnet committees to share knowledge and ideas
- Assigns accountability expectations to other committees
- Reviews and edits documentation submitted by forces committees
- Communicates with hospital leadership and medical staff
- Evaluates progress according to organizational timeline
- Networks with community resources
- Oversees all committees
- Coordinates requests for information or support from other departments
- Coordinates documents for the site visit

Key points for organizational success

Teamwork, patience, dedication, perseverance, and respect across the organization are integral to success. The responsibility for developing the process and preparing the documentation to obtain Magnet cannot be placed solely on one committee or on the Magnet project coordinator, so before the committees even start their projects, conduct both a team-building session and a brainstorming session to share thoughts and generate creativity.

The goal is for the committee members to work in harmony and accomplish their projects, knowing that organizational resources and assistance are available. Although committee members are responsible for achieving specific outcomes, they should focus on the organization as a whole and remember to maintain an interdisciplinary approach to Magnet as they move forward in their work.

Documentation

Often, the committee that faces the biggest challenge is the Forces of Magnetism committee. Documentation required for Magnet needs to be comprehensive, focused, and detailed, and it must contain supporting evidence and showcase nursing excellence across the organization. The following list highlights some key concepts to guide the writing process:

- The organization needs to determine the process. Will the committee prepare drafts for a "designated writer" to edit into a final document, or will the committee be responsible for the final product?
- Brainstorm practice exemplars before writing them to avoid duplication.
- Ideas should be generated by all members.
- Supporting evidence should be collected by all members.
- Cross reference documents to avoid duplication of supporting evidence.
- Final writing of the narrative supporting the Force(s) should be done by one writer for clarity and consistency. Depending on the process established within the organization, submit to either the Magnet project coordinator or the steering committee for final review.
- Have an outside reviewer edit the final document for grammar, logical flow, and consistency.
- Consider hiring a consultant (as discussed in Chapter 2) to review final documents.

"Create co-chairs who are in charge of maintaining deadlines, organizing incoming information, and overseeing the presentation of the document. We felt that by keeping the overall accountability to two people, things stayed in control. I worked with another hospital who had a larger committee structure with standards divided between 10 different individuals, and things just did not move forward. You need to have one or two people with oversight and tight control. Otherwise, the process can take on a life of its own."

—*Katherine Riley, BSN, RN*

Collecting nursing quality indicators

National Database of Nursing Quality Indicators

As we discussed in Chapter 1, there has been ongoing, systematic research on the relationship between nurse-sensitive quality indicators, registered nurse staffing, and patient outcomes. To support research in this area and to provide individual hospitals with national benchmarking opportunities, the American Nurses Association (ANA) created and developed the National Database of Nursing Quality Indicators (NDNQI) in 1998. The program is part of the ANA's quality initiative and is administered by the University of Kansas School of Nursing. Additional information on the NDNQI can be found at *www.nursingquality.org*. The lists below provide a brief overview of key concepts related to the NDNQI.

Benefits of participation

- Participants receive comparative data for internal quality benchmarking
- Participants contribute to ongoing national research database between nurse staffing and patient outcomes
- Participants receive quarter-by-quarter and unit-by-unit comparisons of nursing care
- Participants receive national comparative data for external benchmarking
- Confidentiality is maintained, only you can see your data, and organizational identity is not disclosed
- Participants receive customized reports, including graphic representation comparing their data to national data from similar-sized hospitals
- More than 500 hospitals now participate in this database
- The yearly participation fee is only $3,500 and is prorated for the first year if the organization is submitting only partial-year data
- There is an online nursing satisfaction survey

(Adapted from *Transforming Data Into Quality Care*, publication of the National Database of Nursing Quality Indicators, 2004.)

Relevance to Magnet

- All hospitals applying for Magnet need to participate in a national database that benchmarks nurse-sensitive quality indicators.

- Once a hospital is awarded Magnet status, ongoing participation is required.

- It is necessary to have submitted and received feedback twice and to have it available for appraiser review.

- When initial data is received, organization can review and initiate practice changes if necessary. Remember, it is what you do with the data that counts.

- For Magnet, the following data must be collected at the unit level and then submitted electronically to the NDNQI:
  - Patient falls
  - Maintenance of skin integrity (pressure ulcers prevalence, pressure ulcers occurrence)
  - Patient satisfaction (with overall care, nursing care, patient education, and pain management)
  - Nursing staff satisfaction
  - Nursing care hours per patient day
  - Skill mix of registered nurse (RN), licensed practice nurse (LPN), and unlicensed staff

- In addition, two of the following nurse-sensitive indicators must be collected at the unit level and be a part of the written narrative submitted to the Magnet Program Office (In the event that these indicators are not applicable to some units, choose appropriate indicators that have been shown to be nurse-sensitive):
  - Length of stay
  - Urinary tract infection
  - Upper gastrointestinal (GI) bleed
  - Pneumonia
  - Shock
  - Cardiac arrest
  - Sepsis
  - Deep vein thrombosis
  - Failure to rescue

- There are specific definitions for these indicators, and the organization must use them for data collection.

(Adapted from *The Magnet recognition program: Recognizing excellence in nursing service, application manual,* 2005 Edition.)

"At UCI Medical Center we have an online event-reporting system. We require the indicators for NDNQI, such as falls and pressure ulcers, to be reported electronically, and the system requires that follow-up be completed and entered as well.

We also do a prevalence study on skin twice a year. This is completed by a team of staff nurses who have been trained and have been doing this for several years now. Our risk management department formats the data for us in a manner compatible with NDNQI. Our staffing data is also electronic, and we worked with finance to produce a report in the same manner."

—**Lisa Reiser, RN, MSN**

When to start?

The time to call the NDNQI for an information package is when you are just starting to think about Magnet. The package contains important information on the collection and submission process, definitions of indicators, fee schedules, deadlines for data submission, a timeframe for receiving results, and a contract for participation.

Obtain this information early so planning can begin. For example, the nurse satisfaction survey is currently limited to 70 hospitals submitting data in the same month, so you need to give yourself extra time in case you cannot get your information submitted in the month that is your first choice. Also, you need to give yourself time to review the first set of data and make practice changes before submitting the second.

The Johns Hopkins Hospital in Baltimore already had a performance improvement program in place that included nursing quality indicators. However, because they used NDNQI as a benchmark for the purposes of the Magnet initiative (and submitted the data quarterly as NDNQI requires), they had to make some modifications to their method of collecting indicators due to the way NDNQI desires data. They had no real problems submitting the data electronically because they are an electronically driven institution, but healthcare in general still lacks integrated databases. This presents universal problems for anyone attempting to get good data.

—**Jane Shivnan, MScN, RN, AOCN**

Points to consider

- Do you currently collect data on these indicators, following the prescribed definitions? If not, how long will it take to start the process, and what resources will be required?

- Changing the definition of how you collect data can take time and energy, so be prepared with your rationale as to why this is integral to Magnet.

- If you need to change definitions, how long will it take?

- A nurse satisfaction survey is offered electronically six times a year. However, the paper version is limited to once a year. How computer-savvy are your nursing staff?

- Does the hospital chief executive officer or risk manager need to review the contract?

- Will your organization require institutional review board approval prior to distribution of the nurse satisfaction survey?

- Who will determine the two nurse-sensitive indicators about which your organization collects unit-level data?

- Who will serve as site coordinator for data collection?

Submitting data electronically can be tedious. Also, it's important to be aware that the formulas used for NDNQI are not the same as those used for other reporting databases. So data (like number of falls) for one database may be different from that for another, such as NDNQI.

—Kim Sharkey, RN, MBA, CNAA, BC

Required organizational infrastructure

- Collaborative process among nursing services, quality, and risk management

- Ease of access to information that is currently collected and stored in other departments

- Defined process for data collection

- Secretarial support to enter organizational data into NDNQI online electronic database

- Enthusiastic staff nurse to oversee the nurse satisfaction survey and encourage participation

- Staff nurse access to computers to submit nurse satisfaction survey online

Electronic, quarterly submission of data (e.g., fall data, NHPPD, RN satisfaction survey results, skin breakdown data) to the NDNQI in the revised format is time-consuming. The department of nursing is training an administrative assistant to help with the data entry and electronic submission to NDNQI.

—Anne Jadwin, RN, MSN, AOCN, CNA

References

American Nurses Credentialing Center (2004), *Magnet recognition program: Recognizing excellence in nursing service, application manual (2005 Edition)*. Washington, DC: American Nurses Credentialing Center.

National Database of Nursing Quality Indicators (NDNQI) (2004). *Transforming data into quality care*. Kansas City, KS.

CHAPTER 5

Conducting your gap analysis

Now that you have made the decision and are committed to achieving Magnet recognition, perform an internal assessment to acknowledge the strengths and weaknesses of your organization, identify needed resources, and come up with a realistic time frame in which to transform weakness into excellence.

Part of the Magnet application process is creating a written narrative to allow appraisers to evaluate how the Forces of Magnetism are integrated into your organizational culture. During the gap analysis, identify supporting evidence that substantiates the existence of each Force within your organization.

The person who performs the gap analysis varies among organizations. It can be done by the chief nurse executive in collaboration with the nursing leadership team, the Magnet project coordinator, or an outside consultant. In some organizations, the steering committee is formed early in the process to evaluate organizational readiness, make recommendations for improvements, and collaborate on the timeline.

The following checklist can be helpful as you start the gap analysis.

Figure 5.1	Gap analysis initial checklist

Organizational assessment and readiness	
Review ANA Web site (*www.nursingworld.org*) for the most current eligibility requirements. Click on the link for the American Nurses Credentialing Center and then click on Magnet Recognition.	
Order a current version of the Magnet application manual to review required demographic and narrative data.	
Have all members of the nursing leadership team and a random sample of staff nurses complete the organizational readiness tool (Figure 2.1 on p. 10). Evaluate and compare results between the two groups.	
If you have not already done so, develop a presentation for senior leadership, members of the medical staff, and the hospital board to obtain their support for the project and perspective on organizational readiness.	
Contact NDNQI for an informational package.	
Obtain a current version of *Scope and Standards for Nurse Administrators,* published by AACN.	
Identify a Magnet project coordinator.	
Review RN turnover and vacancy rate and benchmark to national data.	
Verify the percent of RNs in your organization that have achieved certification.	
Review current employee, patient, and physician satisfaction surveys.	
Staff-nurse assessment and readiness	
Have a random sample of direct care RNs complete the survey (Figure 2.4 on p. 20).	
Refer to the staff nurse self-assessment on the ANCC Web site.	
Evaluate the results of staff nurse surveys.	
Hold meetings with staff nurses to hear their perspective on readiness and incorporate this feedback into practice changes.	
Initiate a request for staff nurses to be part of the Magnet process.	
Encourage nursing leadership and staff nurses to become involved in professional organizations.	

The following tool can be useful in assessing the Forces of Magnetism within your organization. The definitions for the Forces of Magnetism are from the *Magnet recognition program: Recognizing excellence in nursing service, application manual (2005 Edition).*

Figure 5.2

Gap analysis for Forces of Magnetism

Forces of Magnetism	Supporting evidence available? (If no, detailed action plan is required. If yes, go to next column.)	Documents or projects to be used as evidence	How difficult will it be to collect the evidence? (Easy, moderate, or hard.)	Who will be responsible for collecting the evidence?	Action plan (Include resources required to complete and responsible party.)	Time frame
1. Quality of nursing leadership *Knowledgeable, strong, risk-taking nurse leaders who follow an articulated philosophy in the day-to-day operations of the nursing department. Nursing leaders that convey a strong sense of advocacy and support on behalf of the staff.*						
2. Organizational structure *Organizational structures are generally flat, rather than tall, and unit-based decision-making prevails. Strong nursing representation is evident in the organizational committee structure. Executive level nursing leaders serve at the executive level of the organization. The chief nursing officer often reports directly to the chief executive officer.*						
3. Management style *Organization and nursing administrators use a participative management style and incorporate feedback from staff at all levels. Feedback is encouraged and valued and nurses serving in leadership positions are visible, accessible, and committed to communicating to the staff.*						
4. Personnel policies and programs *Salaries and benefits are competitive. Creative flexible staffing models are used and shift rotation is minimized. Personnel policies are created with staff involvement. There are significant opportunities for growth in administrative and clinical areas.*						
5. Professional models of care *Models of care are used that give nurses the responsibility and authority for the provision of direct patient care. Nurses are accountable for their own practices, as well as for the coordination of care.*						

Figure 5.2	Gap analysis for Forces of Magnetism (cont.)

Forces of Magnetism	Supporting evidence available? (If no, detailed action plan is required. If yes, go to next column.)	Documents or projects to be used as evidence	How difficult will it be to collect the evidence? (Easy, moderate, or hard.)	Who will be responsible for collecting the evidence?	Action plan (Include resources required to complete and responsible party.)	Time frame
6. Quality of care *Nurses perceive they provide high-quality patient care. Providing quality care is an organizational priority. Nurses serving in leadership positions are seen as responsible for developing the environment in which high-quality care can be provided.*						
7. Quality improvement *Quality improvement is viewed as educational. Staff nurses participate in the process and view the process as one that improves the quality of care delivered in the organization.*						
8. Consultation and resources *Adequate consultation and human resources are available. Knowledgeable experts, including APNs, are available and used. Peer support is given within and outside the nursing division.*						
9. Autonomy *Nurses are permitted and expected to practice autonomously, consistent with professional standards and independent judgment is expected to be exercised within the context of multidisciplinary approach to patient care.*						
10. Community and the hospital *Community presence is often established through ongoing, long-term outreach programs resulting in the hospital being perceived as a strong, positive, and productive corporate citizen. (Hospitals with a strong community presence are able to recruit and retain nurses).*						

Figure 5.2	Gap analysis for Forces of Magnetism (cont.)

Forces of Magnetism	Supporting evidence available? (If no, detailed action plan is required. If yes, go to next column.)	Documents or projects to be used as evidence	How difficult will it be to collect the evidence? (Easy, moderate, or hard.)	Who will be responsible for collecting the evidence?	Action plan (Include resources required to complete and responsible party.)	Time frame
11. Nurses as teachers *Nurses are permitted and expected to incorporate teaching in all aspects of their practice. Teaching gives nurses a great deal of professional satisfaction.*						
12. Image of nursing *Nurses are viewed as an integral part of the hospital's ability to provide patient care. Services provided by nurses are characterized as essential by other members of the health care team.*						
13. Interdisciplinary relationships *A sense of mutual respect among all disciplines, resulting in positive interdisciplinary relationships.*						
14. Professional development *There are opportunities for competency based clinical advancement, along with resources to maintain competency. Value is placed on personal and professional growth and development. Emphasis is placed on orientation, inservice education, continuing education, formal education, and career development.*						

Be honest and realistic when completing this analysis. If you must make cultural changes, consider what resources are needed and what the time frame involved requires. For example, if staff nurses are not participating on hospital committees, will it take just a phone call to make it happen, or is there a negotiating process required to make such a radical change? See Figure 5.3 for an example of how this gap analysis tool can be used.

Figure 5.3	Example of completed gap analysis

Forces of Magnetism	Supporting evidence available? (If no, detailed action plan is required. If yes, go to next column.)	Documents or projects to be used as evidence	How difficult will it be to collect the evidence? (Easy, moderate, or hard)	Who will be responsible for collecting the evidence?	Action plan (Include resources required to complete and responsible party.)	Time frame
7. Quality improvement *Quality improvement is viewed as educational. Staff nurses participate in the process and view the process as one that improves the quality of care delivered in the organization.*	Yes	• Unit-based quality projects (poster boards) • Staff nurses are members of hospital quality council • Staff nurses involved in unit-based quality projects (can use meeting minutes) • Example of change in practice/policy from a quality project • Staff nurse(s) involvement in evidence-based practice	Easy	• Nurse manager of individual unit to submit meeting minutes reflecting discussion at monthly staff meetings. • Staff nurse(s) on nursing quality council will collect unit-based documentation. • Staff nurse(s) on hospital quality council will provide evidence of inter-disciplinary initiatives and resulting practice change. • Staff nurse will submit evidence-based abstract presented at national nursing conference.		1–2 months

Organizational data readiness

What may seem easy to accomplish can be more difficult and time-consuming than it appears. This is often the case with organizational data. At first glance, you might think it is easy to determine the educational level of registered nurses (RN) at the unit level. However, if this information is only captured on the employee application at the time of hire, how is this information transmitted to the nurse manager? Does the human resource department maintain a demographic database of this type for all of nursing services? If so, how is it updated if an RN transfers to another unit or earns an advanced degree? Who is responsible for updating the database? Use the following tool in Figure 5.4 as a guide for assessment of organizational data readiness.

Figure 5.4	Assessment of organizational demographic data readiness

Required demographic data	Do you currently collect? (Yes/no)	Who collects the data?	Who maintains the database?	Who will be responsible for collecting if not currently collecting?	Who will obtain data from various sources?	Who will enter data from various sources into one document for Magnet?	Time frame
Case mix index per unit							
Total nursing care hours by patient day for each unit							
FTEs at each unit level for RNs, LPNs, CNAs, unit clerks							
Vacancy rate by unit							
Controllable/uncontrollable resignations by unit							
FTEs of other health professionals available to unit (OT, PT, social worker)							
Number of APNs per unit							
Educational level of APNs							
Certifications of APNs							
Educational level of RNs (by unit)							
Certifications of RNs (by unit)							
Educational preparation of nurses in leadership roles							

The 14 Forces of Magnetism

What are the 14 Forces?

The Forces of Magnetism were derived from research conducted in the original Magnet hospitals (McClure, Poulin, Sovie, & Wandelt, 2002). They are the 14 differentiating characteristics that enabled these organizations to recruit and retain nurses. Effective in January 2005, the Forces of Magnetism will replace the Magnet standards and become the framework for documentation submission.

In this chapter, the Forces are defined according to the ANCC's *Magnet Nursing Recognition Program: Recognizing Excellence in Nursing Service Application Manual (2005 edition)*. Following each definition is a list of project types that can illustrate how the Force is integrated into nursing within your organization and practice examples provided by Magnet facilities.

The lists are not meant to be exhaustive, and some ideas can support more than one Force. For example, clinical ladders can be highlighted under personnel policies if there are monetary incentives associated with progress. They also can be discussed under professional models of care or professional development.

1. Quality of nursing leadership

Knowledgeable, strong, risk-taking nurse leaders who follow an articulated philosophy in the day-to-day operations of the nursing department. Nursing leaders that convey a strong sense of advocacy and support on behalf of the staff.

Examples of projects or documents to illustrate quality of nursing leadership

- The chief nurse executive (CNE) reports directly to chief executive officer (CEO) and how this enables the CNE to advocate for staff nurses

- A philosophy of nursing that is grounded in a theoretical framework

- Staff nurse involvement in creating nursing strategic plan or nursing mission statement

- Participation in organization for all nurses at all levels

- Involvement in professional organizations for all nurses at all levels

- Publications for all nurses at all levels

- Good staffing ratios

- CNE facilitation of nursing research and evidence-based practice

- Staff nurse satisfaction data and involvement of staff nurses in the process

"At Medical City Dallas Hospital and The North Texas Hospital for Children, quality of nursing leadership was demonstrated through the educational sessions that nurses in the organization attended that taught the 'Nursing as Caring' philosophy and the 'Caring Model' inservices that teach five caring behaviors that each nurse uses with patients. These behaviors were visible on the unit and in the discussions with nursing staff. The philosophy flows through to our documentation, as on the initial assessment we asked for the patient's preferred name, so that we may use it in a caring way when addressing the patient."

—Cole Edmonson, MS, RN, CHE, CNAA, BC

"Evidence of [the quality of nursing leadership] was throughout the application: a copy of the organization's mission statement and organization chart, the role of the executive nurse, examples of how I (we) influence healthcare in our organization, and the roles we assume.

"They specifically looked to see that I was at the major decision-making tables, such as board meetings, strategic planning, capital and resource allocation, and a 'daily operational meeting,' including major medical staff meetings such as the medical executive committee. They look to see that nursing leadership and nurses were on all major (and minor) hospital and medical staff committees. They essentially wanted to see that nursing was at the large and small tables.

"They were very impressed with our shared governance and our collaborative practice environment—that it was in place and not in theory. They looked to see that nurse leaders and staff influence decision-making on patient care. They reviewed my CV and educational attendance and sought examples of how I influenced and/or provided leadership for nursing in the organization. They looked to see the other boards and roles I filled in community service (e.g., March of Dimes, Women in Healthcare, CT Quality Council, etc.).

"We produced a grid that all the directors, managers, and I completed that listed our credentials, that we are certified in nursing administration through ANA, what boards we are on, and what publications and presentations we gave over the last three years—they wanted recent material but did take some history as well.

"They looked to see what we were doing from a quality improvement perspective, what the results of our outcome indicators were, and that we were benchmarking with ANA and have been since it started in 1997. We provided evidence on how I [ensure that] the budget/resources are available for patient care and safe staffing, that there are qualified nurse leaders on patient care units, and that all nurses report, professionally and/or administratively, to me. I demonstrated how I changed our half-time unit managers to full-time and how I enhanced the nurse staffing ratios when patient care demonstrated this need.

"They also wanted to see such things as whether I influence staff to take advantage of educational opportunities; while they were interested in the courses offered, they wanted the attendance sheets of this. They looked at what I was doing to create evidence-based practice and my leadership role in our Capital Area Alliance for Nursing Research and Research Utilization. They check to see how much of this was in place and asked the staff to verify, clarify, and substantiate this—not just the nurse leaders, who all went through an intensive interview. They looked at my leadership in forming a strong partnership with area nursing schools and nursing students and interviewed all the schools we did work with and a sample of their students. They also did the same with key nursing organizations, such as the Connecticut Nurses Association."

—*Laura Caramanica, RN, PhD*

2. Organizational structure

Organizational structures are generally flat, rather than tall, and unit-based decision-making prevails. Strong nursing representation is evident in the organizational committee structure. Executive level nursing leaders serve at the executive level of the organization. The chief nursing officer (CNO) often reports directly to the CEO.

Examples of projects or documents to illustrate organizational structure

- Organizational chart for nursing
- Staff nurse involvement in organizational meetings and interdisciplinary hospital committees
- Shared governance structure in place
- Staff nurse involvement in decision-making, as evidenced by participation in quality, education, leadership, research, practice, recruitment, and retention councils
- Unit-based advisory council
- Minutes of committee and unit meetings reflecting staff nurse participation in organizational decision making

"Our nursing organizational structures are flat, with the clinical managers directly reporting to the CNO. We have a department-wide shared governance model, with unit-based decision-making. Our nursing department is decentralized, and we have strong nursing representation throughout the organization's committee structures. The nursing leader serves at the executive level of the organization."

—Joanne Hambleton, RN, MSN, CNA

"[Our organizational structure] was demonstrated through the organizational chart and meetings with the board of trustees that described the role of the nurse executive as a member of the senior management team, reporting to the CEO, and as actively attending the board. In addition, we shared our participative leadership model of unit-based councils, of which the surveyors attended meetings that were scheduled during the survey time. The hospital committee structure was shared in both policy and diagrams, which demonstrated nursing on each committee as a voting member."

—Cole Edmonson, MS, RN, CHE, CNAA, BC

3. Management style

Organization and nursing administrators use a participative management style and incorporate feedback from staff at all levels. Feedback is encouraged and valued. Nurses serving in leadership positions are visible, accessible, and committed to communicating to the staff.

Examples of projects or documents to illustrate management style

- Unit-based governance councils
- Peer evaluations
- Round-the-clock forum where staff nurses can meet with the CNE to share ideas
- Staff nurse attendance at director/manager meeting
- Staff nurse presentation of practice examples (e.g., small story in which nursing made a difference in a patient's life) at board of trustees or executive team meeting
- Minutes of staff meetings reflecting staff nurse input and feedback to guide clinical decision making

"We embrace a fully integrated participative management style that incorporates feedback from staff at all levels of the organization. Feedback is an important value in communication and the decision-making properties of our organization. Nursing leaders are visible, accessible, and committed to fostering strong communication between leaders and staff throughout the organization. This is demonstrated through our shared governance councils and structures and our quarterly open forums where staff, the CNO, and nursing directors discuss issues of relevance for the department. Minutes from these meetings are sent to all staff."

—Joanne Hambleton, RN, MSN, CNA

"[Our management style] was demonstrated through the sharing of e-mails that occurred between nursing leadership and staff, meeting minutes [for meetings at] which staff were present, the nursing newsletter, CNO lunches with all levels of nursing, and direct questioning of the staff by the surveyors."

—Cole Edmonson, MS, RN, CHE, CNAA, BC

4. Personnel policies and programs

Salaries and benefits are competitive. Creative flexible staffing models are used and shift rotation is minimized. Personnel policies are created with staff involvement. There are significant opportunities for growth in administrative and clinical areas.

Examples of projects or documents to illustrate personnel policies and programs

- Student nurse extern program
- New graduate nurse internship
- Employee advisory committee
- Flexible scheduling options (e.g., Baylor, summers-off program)
- Unit-based self-scheduling
- Differential for certification and educational advancement
- Use of tuition reimbursement dollars to cover the cost of certification
- Retention incentives for employees
- Flexible schedules for employees returning to school
- Administrative mentorship programs

"We are committed to having competitive salaries and benefits. We have established a committee of representatives from human resources, nursing, and marketing who meet on a regular basis to review retention and recruitment strategies. Market comparisons are done two times a year to maintain competitive salaries. Nurse staffing and schedules are designed to be flexible in meeting patient care and staff needs. Staff nurses are actively involved and engaged in clinical promotion activities through our clinical ladder program, administrative policy development, our shared governance structures, and unit- and organization-wide programs and activities."

—Joanne Hambleton, RN, MSN, CNA

5. Professional models of care

Models of care are used that give nurses the responsibility and authority for the provision of direct patient care. Nurses are accountable for their own practice, as well as for the coordination of care.

Examples of projects or documents to illustrate professional models of care

- Registered nurse (RN)/licensed practice nurse (LPN) collaboration
- RN/certified nursing assistant (CNA) model of care
- Model of care that uses nursing theory as a framework
- Career ladders
- Peer- and self-evaluation in place

"Our shared-governance model has staff nurses as members and a staff nurse as the chair. Each unit has a unit clinical improvement committee (UCIC), which has a representative of all job (titles) and shifts as well as support-department representatives. They make decisions about the patient care on that particular unit. The physicians that have patients on the unit then meet with the chair of the UCIC, nursing leaders, and support-department representatives in a forum called Joint Practice. The decisions from UCIC are approved at that level.

"Sometimes the decisions made at UCIC need to go house-wide. Then the UCIC chair would take the recommendations for house-wide implementation to the clinical practice council, which makes clinical decisions that include development and maintenance of policies/procedures for the nursing division. Also, when our medical executive committee has policies that are to be implemented, they are sent to clinical practice, so the nurses determine the next steps."

—Elizabeth Warden, RN, CNA, MS

"Our professional practice model values the support of the role of the registered nurse as the clinical leader with the responsibility and authority to plan and coordinate care in a primary team model of care delivery and collaborative practice. Nurses have accountability [for] their own practice and responsibility for their clinical competence through our clinical-ladder program and our shared-governance model. Nurses have the accountability and responsibility to determine standards of practice to govern the quality of nursing care. In addition, we incorporate staff nurses into administrative decision-making through committee and council authorities."

—Joanne Hambleton, RN, MSN, CNA

6. Quality of care

Nurses perceive they provide high-quality patient care. Providing quality care is an organizational priority. Nurses serving in leadership positions are seen as responsible for developing the environment in which high-quality care can be provided.

Examples of projects or documents to illustrate quality of care

- Results of National Database of Nursing Quality Indicators (NDNQI) benchmarking
- Results of nurse-sensitive indicators
- Results of patient, nurse, and employee satisfaction surveys
- Results from the most recent Joint Commission on Accreditation of Healthcare Organization (JCAHO) survey
- Awards received by the organization
- Nursing leadership and staff nurse involvement in hospital quality initiative
- Staff nurse input into quality measures
- Patient safety initiatives
- Collaborative projects with ethics committee
- Cultural diversity workshops
- Evidence-based nursing projects
- Active nursing research studies
- Minutes of nursing research council

"Our nurses perceive that they are providing high-quality care as demonstrated by high scores in this area on satisfaction surveys. Providing quality care is seen as an organization-wide priority and an intrinsic value to all members of the Center. Nursing leaders at Fox Chase Cancer Center are viewed as responsible for developing environments where high-quality care is provided. The CNO has the authority and influence to design and implement programs that support excellence in patient care and foster nursing excellence through ongoing education programs, advancement opportunities, and recognition programs."

—Joanne Hambleton, RN, MSN, CNA

SURE model—"The SURE nursing professional practice model provides the governance structure for nursing practice at TCH. It is designed to encourage sharing of information and shared decision-making, utilization of effective and efficient resources, recognition and reward of nursing members, and enhancement of cost-effective quality care, service, and work life."

—Jody Childs, MBA, RN

7. Quality improvement

Quality improvement is viewed as educational. Staff nurses participate in the process and view the process as one that improves the quality of care delivered in the organization.

Examples of projects or documents to illustrate quality improvement

- Unit-based quality projects (staff-nurse driven)
- Active involvement of nurse practice or nurse quality council in implementing change based on results of quality improvement projects or NDNQI results
- Unit story boards or posters
- Quality projects are evidence-based and result in change in practice (e.g., include review of the nursing literature)
- Collaboration (interdisciplinary) on hospital-wide quality projects that resulted in change in practice

"Quality improvement and performance management are viewed as educational activities and are inherently important to maintaining quality care throughout our organization. Staff nurses participate in performance improvement activities and perceive these processes as contributing to improvement initiatives in their organizations."

—Joanne Hambleton, RN, MSN, CNA

"[Quality improvement] was demonstrated in the actual site visit by having the surveyors attend a scheduled meeting of a nursing performance improvement (PI) group, [which] reviewed data and made recommendations in the meeting. The nursing staff were also able to speak to their role in PI and the improvements they had seen or been a part of that related to the process. Every nursing area produced a poster of what made their unit Magnet quality, the majority of which contained the PI process in the content."

—*Cole Edmonson, MS, RN, CHE, CNAA, BC*

8. Consultation and resources

Adequate consultation and human resources are available. Knowledgeable experts, including advanced practice nurses, are available and used. Peer support is given within and outside the nursing division.

Examples of projects or documents to illustrate consultation and resources

- Advanced practice nurse (APN)/clinical nurse specialist (CNS) available for nursing consultation
- Staff nurse member of hospital ethics committee
- Ethics committee members available for consultation
- Resources (i.e., journals, library, computer programs) available to support nursing research
- Faculty members available for clinical or research consultation
- Staff nurses and nursing faculty collaboration on research projects
- Educational lunch-and-learns for staff nurses, provided by APNs
- Members of nursing research council available for mentoring or consultation
- Proposal(s) reviewed by nursing research council
- Internal or external funding received to support nursing research initiatives

"We recognize the need to support patient care through having advanced-practice nurses and nursing clinical experts available for staff nurses to provide advice and support in handling clinical and human resources issues. These experts include nurse practitioners, clinical nurse specialists, specially trained pain-resources nurses, masters-prepared clinical managers and directors, as well as peer support from nurses and other disciplines who have gained expert-level knowledge to assist in care planning and coordination."

—Joanne Hambleton, RN, MSN, CNA

"There is an availability of knowledgeable experts, such as clinical nurse specialists, specialty clinicians, care coordinators, and patient care facilitators for peer support and consultation within and outside [of] the nursing division."

—Patricia Collins, RN, MSN, AOCN

9. Autonomy

Nurses are permitted and expected to practice autonomously, consistent with professional standards and independent judgment is expected to be exercised within the context of multidisciplinary approach to patient care.

Examples of projects or documents to illustrate autonomy

- Policies and procedures are evidence-based and reflect professional nursing organization standards
- Staff nurses are active members of the interdisciplinary team
- The nurse practice council is staff nurse–driven
- Staff nurses make unit-based decisions concerning clinical care (e.g., ICU nurses decide on 24-hour visiting hours or to have family members stay in the room during a code)
- Staff nurses have input into products purchased for use in the clinical areas
- Pain management guidelines are evidence-based and staff nurse–driven

"The Professional Nursing Staff (PNS) Organization is the shared governance structure for the nursing staff at Rush University Medical Center. Established in 1983, PNS is an organization of all registered professional nurses, including nurses in management positions, employed by the medical center. Its goals are to provide quality nursing care for patients, promote high levels of professional performance among nurses, establish standards of clinical practice, and monitor nursing practice through peer review. The PNS establishes standards of clinical practice through various standing committees, including the nursing standards of practice (NSP) committee, the nursing standards of care (NSOC) committee, and the nursing documentation committee (NDC).

"The NSP committee consists of nurse representatives from each clinical department who meet monthly. The committee guides the development, implementation, and monitoring of nursing standards of practice. The goal is to annually review and recommend revisions, as necessary, to all nursing policies and procedures to ensure that they reflect current practice standards and guidelines.

"The committee also communicates with clinical areas and identifies education needs regarding new and revised standards. The committee members, who decide [whether] a content expert's review is needed, coordinate the policy review. If necessary, the policy is sent out to the content expert, such as a clinical specialist, for review. Otherwise, a committee member, who refers to current literature and/or current reference books to verify its accuracy, reviews the policy.

"The chair of the NSP committee also sits on the hospital-wide interdisciplinary operational policy and procedure committee to ensure continuity with other medical center policies.

"The NSOC committee is composed of staff nurses representing all departments in nursing. The NSOC committee is responsible for reviewing and revising the current standards of care and for developing additional standards. Standards of care are reviewed at least every two years to ensure [that] they are consistent with current literature. The committee is responsible for communicating with the clinical areas regarding the nursing standards of care.

"The NDC of the PNS is responsible for overseeing nursing documentation. The committee develops and revises nursing forms based on input of staff nurses and in response to performance trends, regulations, policies, and other data. The committee is responsible for streamlining forms so staff can efficiently document completely and accurately. The committee works with many interdisciplinary groups to revise, delete, and create forms and to ensure compliance with regulations. The chair of the documentation committee also sits on the medical records committee of the medical staff."

—Beverly Hancock, MS, RN

"Autonomy for nursing practice at Hartford Hospital (HH) is best exemplified in our nursing shared governance. Council chairs for practice, education, and performance improvement and their members have authority, responsibility, and accountability for their council's work and those governing the professional practice of nursing, including appropriate delegation to unlicensed personnel. Autonomy is self-governance and it is part of being a professional group. Our nurses engage in peer review and also are assisted in preceptor and mentoring programs.

"These are nursing orders for our patient care units that enable nurses to work within their scope of practice, with the full support and consent of our medical staff. Such orders include changes in vital sign frequency, advancement of mobilization, and diet and selected medication that have been reviewed by our pharmacy department for each patient.

"Nursing is a well-respected discipline at HH, and our advance practice nurses/acute care nurse practitioners (APRN/ACNP) provide direct care to patients 24/7 in all of our intensive care units. One would get the sense that the nurse at HH feels they have control of their practice to provide patient care and are encouraged to think and act accordingly. The long ago bureaucracy of chain of command whereby a nurse needed to ask for even the simplest of orders to a nurse manager or supervisor no longer dictates practice."

—Laura Caramanica, RN, PhD

"Demonstrable aspects of [autonomy] included policy/procedures being based on the nurse practice act to the fullest extent, and included the national organizations standards such as [those of] AORN, AACN, ANA, etc. The policies reflect the actual verbiage from the standards, and nursing staff are all educated on the content, intent, and application of the policy. Nursing role and decision [-making] authority is clearly outlined in programs, chain of command, and policy and procedures that govern patient care. Nursing is considered to be the coordinator of care as well as the hands-on care provider as defined by our scope of practice document and policy and procedures."

—Cole Edmonson, MS, RN, CHE, CNAA, BC

10. Community and the hospital

Community presence is often established through ongoing, long-term outreach programs, resulting in the hospital being perceived as a strong, positive, and productive corporate citizen. (Hospitals with a strong community presence are able to recruit and retain nurses.)

Examples of projects or documents to illustrate community and the hospital

- List of professional organizations to which nurses (including nurse leaders and staff nurses) belong
- Grid showing leadership roles of nurses in local, regional, or national professional organizations
- List of all presentations at local, regional, and national professional conferences
- Involvement of nurses in state nursing associations
- List of all publications by members of the nursing staff
- Involvement of nurses in community events
- Volunteer activities of the nursing staff
- Philanthropic support for nursing projects
- Relationships with local schools or colleges of nursing
- Hospital involvement in community organizations

"We have designed strong connections to the community through our network affiliation programs. These partnerships serve and maintain a presence through a variety of ongoing community-focused activities. Outreach programs, continuing education programs, consultations, and meetings are present in the network program to ensure strong partnerships and positive corporate citizenship activities and outcomes."

—Joanne Hambleton, RN, MSN, CNA

"Community presence is established though active involvement in community activities and ongoing, long-term outreach programs resulting in our hospital being perceived as a strong, positive, and productive corporate citizen."

—Patricia Collins, RN, MSN, AOCN

11. Nurses as teachers

Nurses are permitted and expected to incorporate teaching in all aspects of their practice. Teaching gives nurses a great deal of professional satisfaction.

Examples of projects or documents to illustrate nurses as teachers

- Staff nurses serve as mentors, preceptors, or adjunct faculty members
- Preceptor program that is in place
- Examples of patient education strategies that are in place (e.g., videos, brochures)
- Active involvement of family members in nurses' teaching
- Community educational programs that are supported by the hospital
- Interdisciplinary approach to patient teaching
- Guest lectures done by staff nurses for community agencies

"Nurses are permitted, and expected, to integrate teaching in all aspects of their patient care activities. This integrated practice is perceived by our nurses as one of the activities that provides a high level of professional satisfaction within their roles as staff nurses. Staff nurses are members of our continuing education faculty programs, providing presentations related to their areas of expertise and interest. Fox Chase nurses present in national conferences and in national professional publications."

—Joanne Hambleton, RN, MSN, CNA

"Texas Children's nurses are actively involved in the education of nurses and other professions. Affiliation agreements exist with 13 area schools of nursing, which accounts for the education of [more than] 400 students annually."

—Jody Childs, MBA, RN

"Nurses are permitted and expected to incorporate teaching in all aspects of their practice. Numerous patient education resources are available to assist the nurse with patient education. Nurses are also permitted and expected to teach share their knowledge and expertise with their peers."

—Patricia Collins, RN, MSN, AOCN

---

12. Image of nursing

Nurses are viewed as an integral part of the hospital's ability to provide patient care. Services provided by nurses are characterized as essential by other members of the healthcare team.

Examples of projects or documents to illustrate image of nursing

- Link to nursing Web page from hospital home page
- Biosketch of nurse leaders and select staff nurses on nursing Web page
- Awards won by staff nurses
- Nurse involvement in interdisciplinary patient-centered organizational committees

"[This is] demonstrable by nonnursing members that participated in the survey and documentation process, such as medical staff leadership, community leaders, board of trustees members, and ancillary providers that offered anecdotal examples of nursing contribution. The image of nursing was easily demonstrable through the reward and recognition systems for both individual and group awards. Nurses are celebrated and recognized by peers and nonnursing peers in forums such as leadership meetings, board meetings, and external recognition events in the community."

—Cole Edmonson, MS, RN, CHE, CNAA, BC

"The image of nursing is really a reflection of how nurses see themselves and their professionmore than anything else. Upon interview, Magnet examiners would listen to the words that nurses used and look for evidence that they felt empowered to practice according to the way they feel they were taught and to meet patient needs. Signs of hopelessness and helplessness or horizontal disagreements do not fill the practice environment. How nurses dress, hold their heads, and conduct themselves portrays their confidence in their abilities and their right place at the point of service/care.

"At Hartford Hospital, one is able to see nurses attending treatment rounds and educational rounds and participating, including initiating discussion and giving advice—not just providing information or seeking guidance. Nurses are a part of every service team's healthcare team (i.e., interdisciplinary team that develops and administers to all clinical guidelines and evidence-based practice).

"Nursing, particularly the practicing nurse, is on every hospital and medical committee where patient care or some aspect of patient care, such as materials management/product evaluation, is discussed and planned for. The chief nursing officer sits on the hospital's governance and is instrumental in the decisions affecting all of the hospital's operations, including but not limited to patient care. It is without question that nursing is a vital link to the quality of patient care, and nurses in all roles through the organization are answerable to those outcomes and respected for their contributions. There is evidence of tangible means of rewarding and recognizing nursing staff at Hartford Hospital."

—*Laura Caramanica, RN, PhD*

13. Interdisciplinary relationships

A sense of mutual respect among all disciplines, resulting in positive interdisciplinary relationships.

Examples of projects or documents to illustrate interdisciplinary relationships:

- Nurse-physician round tables, grand rounds, lunch-and-learns
- Results of nurse-physician relationship survey
- Nurse physician collaboration on patient-focused committees
- Interdisciplinary quality projects
- Interdisciplinary research projects

"The ICU units implemented daily multidisciplinary rounds in September of 2002 with the goals of improving communication among different disciplines and setting realistic, attainable goals for patients.

"Participants include nurses, physicians, pharmacists, respiratory therapists (RT), care managers, and dieticians. A brief summary of the patient's progress is given, medications are reviewed, and all participants decide on the patient's goal for that day. Some of the outcomes seen thus far include inappropriate or unnecessary medications are minimized by reviewing the patient's current drug regimen on a daily basis; ventilator weaning is expedited when RTs and RNs clearly communicate the need to minimize sedation and all are working toward that goal; therapies are implemented earlier to prevent complications (like deep vein thrombosis in the immobile patient); end-of-life issues are addressed and code status decisions made more appropriately; and discharge planning is implemented much faster, addressing issues such as long-term IV access, long-term care placement, etc.

"We have seen this process [ensure] organized, systematic care in the ICUs, with more efficient and timely delivery of care. There is shared decision-making among the disciplines, with everyone's expertise valued. The rounds have been so successful that they have now been implemented on all patient care units."

—Sherill Nones Cronin, PhD, RN, BC

"The documentation in the patient record and meeting minutes highlighted not only the leadership of nursing but the coordination of resources and the collaborative relationship that exists in the patient care process."

—Cole Edmonson, MS, RN, CHE, CNAA, BC

"Nursing works closely with many other disciplines and departments to provide excellent patient care. One example is the work of an interdisciplinary team related to a special population. In response to a rising number of bariatric patients admitted to the medical center and the unique challenges associated with their care, an interdisciplinary committee was formed to explore the care of the bariatric patient.

"The team was lead by a nurse manager and consisted of dieticians, engineers, pharmacists, physicians, nurses, and staff from purchasing. After researching the literature and calling other facilities, the team developed a critical pathway for care. This pathway was reviewed and approved by the surgical quality improvement committee, pharmacy and therapeutics committee, and the medical care evaluation committee, which are all interdisciplinary committees.

"The bariatric care team also led staff and patient evaluations of bariatric equipment, which was then purchased, and they developed a flow chart for use of the bariatric beds. They also created patient education for the gastric bypass patients. Finally, they identified the need for and hired new assistive personnel, specifically trained to help with lifting to reduce the burden on the nursing staff. The work of this team provided the nursing staff with needed equipment, information, and support to care for this challenging patient population."

—Beverly Hancock, MS, RN

"Hartford Hospital exemplifies collaborative practice through the entire healthcare setting. In 1992, the hospital participated in a five-year grant from the Robert Wood Johnson and Pew Memorial Trust to strengthen hospital nursing, and from that grant came the redesign of patient care leading up to Collaborative Practice Teams [Nurse/Physician Dyads] that serve as clinical and managerial leadership for all specialties [women's health services, cancer care, surgical services, etc.]. The CMT provides leadership for the healthcare teams [HCTs] that are an interdisciplinary team of licensed providers [nurses, pharmacists, dietary, respiratory therapy, PT/OT, etc.]. The HCT works together to plan, develop, revise, evaluate, and implement all treatment protocols and unit or service operations. The nurse executive and the VP for medical staff affairs are considered the executive CMTs and meet quarterly with CMTs to develop, plan, and evaluate service-wide/specialty-specific goals, keeping these aligned with the hospital's strategic plan and with measurable outcomes. A book was produced describing this (patient care) model: *Collaborative Practice at Hartford Hospital*. It was published through the American Hospital Association in the mid-1990s. Many medical and hospital staff committees are co-led by a nurse and physician or nurse and other discipline such as pharmacist, respiratory therapist, etc. It is important to point out that the practicing nurse serves in many key leadership roles in patient care, and not just nurse managers/educators/clinical nurse specialists."

—Laura Caramanica, RN, PhD

14. Professional development

There are opportunities for competency-based clinical advancement, along with resources to maintain competency. Value is placed on personal and professional growth and development. Emphasis is placed on orientation, inservice education, continuing education, formal education, and career development.

Examples of projects or documents to illustrate professional development

- On-site RN-BSN completion program
- Career (clinical) ladders
- Web-based tutorials
- Career development for LPNs, CNAs, and unit clerks
- Certification review courses on site
- On-site CEU classes
- Competency-based orientation
- Presence of career-development counselor
- Inservice opportunities for weekends and off-shift nurses
- Nursing excellence awards
- Continuing education activities of nurses in leadership roles
- Integration of cultural competency into continuing education programs

"We place a significant emphasis on orientation, inservices, continuing education, formal education, and career development. Professional growth and development are valued, as are opportunities for competency-based clinical advancement and clinical competency. Our nurse continuing education program has a regional reputation for excellence. Our clinical ladder program includes five levels of advancement for staff nurses, three levels for LPN, and three levels for CNAs. We emphasize and support lifelong learning as a way to ensure clinical competence and reward professional development. This is supported through tuition reimbursement, funding for conference attendance for staff nurses, and scholarship programs for staff nurses."

—Joanne Hambleton, RN, MSN, CNA

EXCEL+ Program: "The clinical and professional development program for RNs recognizes nurses' involvement in professional organizations and community-based groups. It also places emphasis on staff teaching and participation on special projects, task forces, research, publishing, etc."

—Jody Childs, MBA, RN

"All RNs promoted to leadership positions attend a 30-hour 'Transition to Leadership' course to assist in their leadership development. We have a tuition reimbursement program to encourage LPN to RN, and RN to BSN and MSN. We reimburse for certification. In addition, staff RNs are encouraged to attend the leadership course to let them explore the possibility of moving to a leadership position. We are also a New York State Nurses Association continuing education (CE) provider and provide a variety of on-site CE programs."

—Diane Peyser, RN, MS, BC, CNA

References

American Nurses Credentialing Center (2004). *Magnet recognition program: Recognizing excellence in nursing service application manual (2005 Edition)*. Washington, DC: American Nurses Credentialing Center.

McClure, M., Poulin, A., Sovie, M., & Wandelt, M. (2002). Magnet hospitals: Attraction and retention of professional nurses (the original study). In M. McClure & A. Hinshaw (Eds.), *Magnet hospitals revisited: Attraction and retention of professional nurses* (pp. 1–24). Washington, DC: American Nurses Publishing.

Crosswalking Magnet criteria to JCAHO standards

Relationship of Magnet to the JCAHO

Recently, the Joint Commission on Accreditation of Healthcare Organizations (JCAHO) acknowledged the value of Magnet designation in resolving the nursing crisis and ensuring high standards for patient safety and quality of care. Currently, surveyors use tracer methodology to survey organizations: they select a patient and use that individual's record to trace or follow the patient through the continuum of care. Doing so gives surveyors the opportunity to assess and evaluate the standards for providing care and the services within the organization.

Along the way, surveyors will observe and talk to staff. The JCAHO announced that beginning in January 2006, all regular accreditation surveys will be unannounced. This change was made to allow surveyors the opportunity to observe performance under normal circumstances and to keep the focus on providing high-quality care at all times. For some organizations, this new lack of warning may result in a feeling of unpreparedness.

However, the good news for organizations is that preparing for, achieving, and sustaining Magnet status is extremely beneficial when it comes to preparing for the JCAHO. Magnet and the JCAHO are complementary in many ways. The following table identifies similarities between the two accreditations.

Figure 7.1	Magnet and JCAHO similarities

J
C
MAGNET
H
O

- Organizations pay a fee to apply for JCAHO accreditation and Magnet recognition.

- Both the JCAHO and Magnet involve two- to three-day surveys or site visits.

- Appraisers from both the JCAHO and Magnet focus their discussions on employees providing direct patient care.

- Organizations must demonstrate adherence to rigorous standards.

- They are interested in best practices, benchmarking quality data, nurse staffing ratios, and environment of care.

- They review policies and procedures in terms of being evidence-based, current, and relevant to practice.

- Professional development is valued; employee files may be reviewed during site visit.

- Ongoing surveys are required to maintain accreditation. Magnet recognition is granted for four years; regular JCAHO surveys occur every three years.

- Either's decision can be revoked if the organization fails to maintain standards.

- Consumers can report issues of concern, which will be investigated during the site visit.

The JCAHO benefits of preparing for and sustaining Magnet

Preparing for and sustaining Magnet will help organizational readiness for unannounced JCAHO surveys. Consider the following benefits:

- Policy and procedures will be organized, current, relevant, and evidence-based.
- Intense dialogue with Magnet appraisers increases the confidence of staff nurses when communicating with JCAHO surveyors.
- Culture of interdisciplinary teamwork, respect, and organizational pride is fostered and maintained.
- Organizational databases are reviewed and updated.
- Participation in national benchmarking database allows for ongoing monitoring.
- Practice is continually evaluated and changed based on empirical evidence.
- Interdisciplinary collaboration is increased.
- Departmental networking evolves.
- Quality improvement projects are staff nurse–driven.

Collaboration with quality department

Often, the quality department of an organization is responsible for regulatory overview, compliance issues, and collection of relevant benchmarking data. Magnet provides an excellent opportunity for collaboration between the quality department and nursing services.

Staff nurses can be members of regulatory review task forces, conduct mock surveys to ensure JCAHO readiness, and assist in the collection and analysis of national benchmarking data. In turn, the quality staff can assist in collection of data for the NDNQI and provide mentorship to staff nurses as they prepare for the site visit.

The following is an example of a crosswalk among the 2003-04 Magnet standards, the 2004 JCAHO standards and the 2005 Magnet Forces of Magnetism. Starting in January 2005, organizations applying for Magnet will use the Forces of Magnetism as the framework for document submission (ANCC, 2004).

Figure 7.2	Magnet crosswalk

2003–04 Magnet standards	2004 JCAHO standards	2005 Forces of Magnetism
Assessment **1.1 Identifies assessment elements including nurse-sensitive quality indicators appropriate to a given organizational context.** Narrative: A statement that best illustrates how your organization meets this criterion in a way that is innovative, dynamic, and incorporates the Forces of Magnetism. Include supporting documentation that best substantiates the narrative. Evidence: • A copy of the healthcare organization's mission statement • A copy of the nursing philosophy • A copy of the organizational chart • A copy of nursing's continuous quality improvement plan. (Evidence of participation in the American Nurses Association's nursing-sensitive quality indicators project) • Other applicable evidence of compliance with this standard	Nursing: NR.1.10-NR.1.10 Elements of Performance 1 Improving Organizational Performance: LD.4.10-LD.4.20 and PI.1.10-PI.3.10	**Force 5: Professional models of care** Expectation: There are models of care that give nurses the responsibility and authority for the provision of direct patient care. Nurses are accountable for their own practice as well as the coordination of care. The models of care (i.e., primary nursing, case management, family-centered, district, and holistic) provide for the continuity of care across the continuum. The models take into consideration patients' unique needs and provide skilled nurses and adequate resources to accomplish desired outcomes. Evidence: • State Nurse Practice Act and other regulatory and professional standards are available as references on each unit and incorporated into practice decisions • Evidence that the continuity of care is addressed in the professional model(s) for the delivery of care • A copy of the scheduling and staffing plan for each unit **Force 6: Quality of care** Expectation: Quality is the systematic driving force for nursing and the organization. Nurses serving in leadership positions are responsible for providing an environment that positively influences patient outcomes. Evidence: • Evidence that direct care nurses perceive that they are providing high-quality patient care • Evidence of how each step of the nursing process is carried out in nursing practice throughout the organization • Evidence that patient safety/quality initiatives have been developed, implemented, and evaluated by nurses at all levels **Force 7: Quality improvement** Expectation: The organization has structures and processes for the measurement of quality and programs for improving the quality of care and services within the organization. Evidence: • A copy of the organization's quality plan • Evidence that the process and rationale for the identification, development, and utilization of national databases that include nursing-sensitive measures that impact patient outcomes

Figure 7.2	Magnet crosswalk (cont.)

1.3 Monitor and evaluate assessment processes that are sensitive to the unique and diverse needs of individuals and target populations.

Narrative: A statement that best illustrates how your organization meets this criterion in a way that is innovative, dynamic, and incorporates the Forces of Magnetism. Include supporting documentation that best substantiates the narrative.

Evidence:

- Assessment of the population the healthcare organization serves
- Definition of special populations by percentage of total population served
- A sample of an educational program conducted to educate nursing staff on cultural competencies and/or special population-specific skills or comparable evidence

Leadership:
LD.3.10, LD.4.20, PI.1.10

Assessment:
PC.2.120-PC.16.60, IM.6.30, LD.3.10, LD.3.50, PC.2.20, MS.2.20, PC.2.120, PC.2.130, PC.2.150

Continuum of Care:
PC.1.10-PC.15.30, RI.1.40

Nursing: NR Overview: Assess the patient care needs: NR.1.10-NR.2.10

Care of Patients:
PC.13.30, MM.3.20, MM.4.80, MM.6.10, MM.6.20, MM.8.10, PC.13.20, LD.3.90

Force 5: Professional models of care
Expectation: (see above)
Evidence:
- Evidence that the model of care addresses patient needs, patient population demographics, number of nursing staff members, and ratio of nurses serving in various roles and levels
- Evidence that direct care nurses implement a model of care designed to meet the needs of specific patient populations at the unit level
- Evidence that the scheduling process is tailored to the patient population, unit needs, and the needs of individual staff members

Force 6: Quality of care
Expectation: (see above)
Evidence:
- Examples of programs developed to meet the cultural, ethical, and demographic needs of a diverse patient population and the resources, fiscal and human, allocated to support these programs.
- Evidence that the nursing organization prepares the professional staff to meet the projected needs of diverse populations.
- Copies of policies and procedures that reflect how the organization address patient/resident language and hearing needs.

Force 7: Quality improvement
Expectation: (see above)
Evidence:
- Demonstrate how the chief nursing officer has effectively influenced system-level change to improve the quality of care
- Evidence that nursing services provides the resources, education, and support to facilitate staff involvement in quality improvement activities
- Examples of nurse involvement in evidence-based quality initiatives to improve coordination and delivery of care across the continuum of services

References

Joint Commission on Accreditation of Healthcare Organizations. Retrieved July 18, 2004, from *www.jcaho.org*

The application process

The Magnet phases

The Magnet process can take anywhere from two to four years from idea generation to site visit. It can be challenging to identify projects, stay focused, meet deadlines, and keep energized over this period of time. However, give yourself time to complete each phase without rushing. A major theme from interviews with chief nurse executives (CNE) is that the writing requires a lot more time than expected.

The purpose of this chapter is to identify the phases, provide a list of major projects to accomplish during each phase, and present best practices from Magnet facilities. Again, our assignment of specific tasks to the phases should not be taken as an absolute or followed rigidly. Rather, it is intended to be a guide, and at times there may be overlap. The process consists of four phases (Urden & Monarch, 2002):

- The application phase
- Submission of written document and evaluation phase
- The site visit phase
- Magnet decision phase

From experience, I have found it helpful to add a preplanning phase.

Preplanning phase

This phase starts when the idea for Magnet is generated. It involves assessing organizational readiness, creating methods of communication about Magnet within your organization, conducting an initial gap analysis, and initiating the needed cultural transformations.

Although CNEs of some organizations may have incorporated some of the following tasks into the application phase, remember that the time clock starts when you send in your one-page application and application fee. If you have some of these details finalized or the process in place to finalize, you will be able to dedicate the next 24 months to writing narratives and preparing for the site visit.

Major projects to accomplish

- Order Magnet application manual to review fee structure and eligibility criteria
- Meet with the nursing leadership team to assess organizational readiness
- Review staff nurse involvement in nursing/hospital committee(s)
- Start the dialogue with the executive team
- Organize a presentation on Magnet for staff nurses
- Consider creating a steering committee to assist with evaluating readiness and initiating cultural changes
- Identify a Magnet project coordinator
- Obtain information from the National Database of Nursing Quality Indicators (NDNQI) and begin the enrollment process
- Prepare a tentative budget for Magnet
- Begin thinking about the process in terms of your organization:
    - Do we need additional secretarial support?
    - Will we have one writer and will he/she be internal or external?
    - Will we have multiple writers and one editor?
    - Will we hire an external consultant?
- Organize Magnet teams (e.g., committees, task forces, etc.)
- Attend a Magnet workshop
- Contact or visit a Magnet hospital in your area

Kathryn "Ginger" Ward-Presson, RN, MSN, chief nursing executive and associate director of nursing care at Miami VA Medical Center in Miami, decided to apply for Magnet in the spring of 2004 but is taking 18–24 months to focus on implementing changes before she sends the check and one-page application. "I know I have some work to do, and this planning is part of the process—and then we will be in great shape when we are ready to write our narratives," says Ward-Presson.

The following is a list of projects that Miami VA Medical Center has initiated or will initiate in the next 18–24 months:

- Performed organizational readiness assessment.
- Obtained support from senior leadership, including a three-year budget plan to support Magnet initiatives.
- Held a nursing retreat to discuss the strategic plan for nursing. Invited participants included staff nurses (RNs), licensed practice nurses (LPNs), and nursing assistants.
- Met with nursing leaders and staff nurses to identify the theme, "We are going on a Magnet Safari."
- Hired an external consultant to assist with gap analysis, cultural transformation, and review of written narratives.
- Secured funding from the operational budget to create additional nursing positions, including a nurse researcher (doctoral-prepared), nurse educators, clinical specialists, a nurse recruiter, and recruitment staff.
- Created a new position for Magnet project coordinator.
- Applied for and received a VA grant to support development of a professional practice model.
- Created position of manager of performance improvement and professional practices.
- Began implementation of a nursing practice model grounded in a caring framework (in process).
- Restructured nursing committees to increase staff nurse visibility and participation in clinical decision-making. Committees include education, research, recruitment and retention, and nursing practice and policy (in process).
- Increasing staff nurse participation on hospital committees (in process).

Do not underestimate the effort it takes to organize all of the documentation. Assembling the binders alone takes weeks. The Magnet journey requires an organized, strategic effort. Involve as many people early on as possible to ensure that the application process runs smoothly.

—Barbara Wadsworth, RN, MSN, CNAA

"Use all the information about Magnet available today as an aid while preparing documentation."

—Barbara Wadsworth, RN, MSN, CNAA

"Determine the motives for pursuing this recognition from the very beginning. The pursuit of Magnet must be motivated by a sincere understanding of the value of the employees. They are a necessity to accomplish the goals of the facility. The decision to begin the journey must be prompted by a desire to change the working environment until it is optimal for the employee, thus resulting in less turnover, better patient outcomes, and professional behavior. Any other motivation is a waste of time for the nursing staff."

—Toni Fiore, MA, RN, CNAA

"Strive for an environment of excellence not recognition. Magnet environments positively impact the nursing staff. Make structural and process changes because they are good for the staff, not because an organization seeks national recognition. If staff perceive that a structure is implemented because the organization wants recognition, they will feel alienated and disenchanted. They will not feel valued; they will feel used."

—Beverly Hancock, MS, RN

"Learn from others, but allow your own organization to guide your journey. Your application should reflect the organization's values and work."

—Beverly Hancock, MS, RN

The application phase

This phase starts when the organization sends in the one-page application and an initial fee of $2,500. Please review the Magnet manual for the fee in place at the time of submission. The fee is nonrefundable, and you now have 24 months to send all the written narratives and supporting documents to the Magnet Project Office. On the application, you will need to identify the date on which the organization plans to submit the written documents. At this point, there may be a blending of projects from the preplanning phase, depending on your individual readiness, available resources, and what you have already accomplished.

Major projects to accomplish

- Submit one-page application and check for $2,500 to Magnet Program Office
- Formal presentation on Magnet to key stakeholders (e.g., executive team, board of trustees, physicians)
- Conduct ongoing reviews of organizational and nursing resources, standards, and policies
- Increase organizational (interdisciplinary) awareness and involvement in the process
- Host a kick-off event announcing that the journey has begun to energize the organization
- Formalize steering committee membership
- Assemble Magnet committees and seek additional volunteers if needed
- Submit first set of data to NDNQI
- Network with leaders/staff nurses of other Magnet facilities
- Prepare a timeline
- Identify a Magnet theme

Submission of written document and evaluation phase

This phase involves compiling the written narratives and supporting evidence for submission to the Magnet Program Office and then waiting for the documents to be reviewed by the appraisers. During this phase, the group(s) working on the narratives must stay focused on the details, meet the deadlines, and avoid feeling stressed. Magnet facilities have referred to this phase as "time-consuming," "tedious," "exhausting," "rewarding," "challenging," or "the best experience we have ever had as an organization." The key to success is ongoing support from the CNE and the ability to reprioritize daily activities in order to complete the documents.

Not only do you need to complete the documents, you need to factor in time for quality editing and expert review by an external consultant. Quality editing is especially important if there are multiple writers. The decision to use an external consultant for document review is optional. Note that only 70% of the submitted documents achieve a score in the range of excellence, which is the score needed to have a site visit scheduled by the appraiser team (Romano, 2002).

Prior to compiling and submitting the written documents, please refer to the Magnet manual for specific instructions on the number of binders, use of cross-reference material, font size, and shipping. At this time, documents cannot be transmitted electronically.

Major projects to accomplish

- Written narratives completed and mailed to Magnet Project Office

- All Magnet committees actively engaged in the process and meeting deadlines

- Staff nurses involved in Magnet projects

- Communication process(es) in place to keep all employees updated on the progress

- Community resources (six) identified and have provided a letter of support

- Educational fairs and mock surveys held to prepare for site visit

- Check for appraisal fee is sent in with documents

- All organizational overview and demographic data collected

- Second set of data submitted to NDNQI early in this phase so applicants have two sets of data for appraisers to review

- Site-visit documents organized

"The most important single piece of advice I can give is do not underestimate the amount of time and energy that will be required to write the application." Jadwin says she should have doubled the amount of time designated for writing the narratives in the established timeline and that she could not keep pace with her timelines due to other duties as director of nursing. Eventually, she began setting weekly deadlines, and if she didn't finish all of the tasks she'd assigned herself, she spent time over the weekend catching up.

—*Anne Jadwin, RN, MSN, AOCN, CNA*

Avoiding work on the weekends proved to be a powerful incentive for Jadwin. She booked blocks of writing time (at least two to three hours) because working on narratives for only an hour at a time was unproductive. She also found that forwarding completed narratives to the vice president of nursing for review and editing was helpful. Once the edits were complete, the administrative assistant made copies for the manuals and compiled any necessary sample exhibits. This was important because the department was able to keep up with the workload and not feel overly burdened in the end.

—*Anne Jadwin, RN, MSN, AOCN, CNA*

"Every stage of our process took more time than we predicted, gathering documents, writing the narratives, and organizing the evidence into the narratives. On our original timeline, we planned to have submitted our documentation in January 2004. We finally submitted our bound documents to the ANCC on May 18."

—Norine Watson, RN, MSN, CNA, BC

"Identify one project coordinator to secure a single voice in the documentation. Everyone should contribute to the generation of ideas, but one project manager is essential to the maintenance of organization throughout the Magnet journey."

—Janet Ahlstrom, MSN, RN, BC, M-SCNS

"Host open forums on all units to solicit feedback and stories about how the hospital meets the Magnet standards so that the narrative is a reflection of everyone's input. Put the application (theirs was four binders!) on a 'Magnet cart' for a couple of weeks in each unit so staff can review it."

—Laura Caramanica, RN, PhD

"Instead of assigning standards to various nurse leaders, request outlines of solid evidence of compliance with the standards (programs, care initiatives, etc.). Then, as the Magnet coordinator, take the evidence and write the documents yourself. Too many voices and too much overlap occurred when asking various nurse leaders to write full documents. It is important that all the standards flow with the same voice and use the same syntax and style. I rewrote the majority of the standards from what I was given so that they were consistent."

—Barbara Hannon, MSN, RN

"Have the writers attend a retreat hosted by nursing leadership in which they learn more about the application standards and begin brainstorming about how the facility can offer evidence of compliance with the standards."

—Patricia Collins, RN, MSN, AOCN

The site visit phase

If after review of the documents by the appraisers it has been determined that the score is within the range of excellence, then a site visit is scheduled. The appraisers, who evaluate the documents, conduct the site visit. The site visit is usually two days, but that may vary depending on the size of the organization. Typically, two appraisers conduct the site visit, but larger organizations may require an additional appraiser. During the site visit, the appraisers will meet with the CNE, staff nurses, members of nursing leadership, and members of various nursing or hospital committees. Additionally, appraisers will interview the chief executive officer, the chief operating officer, the chief financial officer, and other interdisciplinary leaders.

Prior to the site visit, you will be required to post formal notices in the organization notifying employees, visitors, consumers, and the local community about the organization's Magnet application and upcoming site visit. The intent is to provide an opportunity for any of the above groups to provide feedback or comments. The Magnet Program Office will provide the specifications concerning placement and content of the public notices.

The purpose of the appraiser's site visit is to evaluate how the Forces of Magnetism are operationalized in the day-to-day management of the organization. Their specific intent is to evaluate, verify, and clarify the written documentation. During the site visit, the appraisers may review a number of documents, including the following:

- Minutes of meetings focused on quality improvement issues for the past 12 months
- All nursing research findings from the past 12 months
- The CNE's educational history over the past year
- Examples of communication between the CNE and nurses who provide direct patient care
- Results of patient, employee, and nurse satisfaction survey(s) for the past 12 months

(Adapted from *The Magnet nursing services recognition program for excellence in nursing service, health care organization, instructions and application process manual,* 2003–2004.)

Appraisers will interview staff nurses during the site visit. Staff nurses generally are very excited to talk about the rewarding experience of the Magnet journey and enjoy sharing examples of excellence in nursing care. They are proud of the care they deliver and of the professional practice environment they work in, so talking with the appraisers is seen as a positive, nonstressful experience. The following are a few examples of the types of questions that may be asked during the site visit.

Questions appraisers may ask during site visit

- Has the CNE been an advocate for nurses?
- Does the formal structure indicate nurse participation at all levels in the development of the budget for the nursing system?
- What is the professional staff nurse-patient ratio at this time?
- Is input from peers incorporated into evaluations of fellow nurses?
- Are there opportunities for flexible/modified schedules?
- Does the nurse representative(s) on the ethic committee(s) have voting privileges?
- Are nursing personnel submitting research proposals to the research committees for review?

(Adapted from *The Magnet nursing services recognition program for excellence in nursing service, health care organization, instructions and application process manual, 2003–2004.*)

Major projects to accomplish

- Coordinate date of site visit and travel arrangements with appraisers
- Display public announcements as required by Magnet Program Office
- Collect and organize all required documents for appraiser(s) to review during site visit
- Hold Magnet fairs and educational sessions for all employees
- Have round-the-clock meetings and mock surveys

In preparation for the site visit, the Magnet project coordinator worked from April to September with staff nurses to "Magnetize the institution." They created a role called the Magnet ambassador—a staff nurse who was selected by peers and represented the unit in Magnet activities (there were 60 at JHH, and some represented more than one unit). Selection as ambassadors had nothing to do with seniority; rather, they were chosen by their colleagues for attributes such as "realistic optimism."

The ambassadors attended a full-day workshop in June, in which they learned about Magnet and shared exemplars. The ambassador role was the main method used to communicate with the various units in the hospital, and Ambassadors worked hard to build knowledge and enthusiasm about Magnet recognition using meetings, games, contests, quizzes, bulletin boards, mock surveys.

Based on an educational Magnet timeline, the ambassadors tackled a new topic every 10 days or so. Ultimately, their task was not educating staff but rather making them comfortable talking about what they already do.

—Jane Shivnan, MScN, RN, AOCN

Have a "Magnet Breakfast of Champions" prior to the site visit to make sure the unit champions are ready for the surveyors and to celebrate their involvement in the process. Provide them with "talking tips" in writing. Conduct mock survey visits to all units to prepare staff.

Host departmental inservices in which the Forces of Magnetism are presented to attendees. Create sample Q & As for the 14 Forces and distribute them to staff members. Have staff move around to various stations and field questions from nursing leaders about the standards.

Send a customized letter to physicians and departments throughout the facility and invite them to attend the drop-in session during the site visit.

—Anne Jadwin, RN, MSN, AOCN, CNA

The decision phase

Following their site visit, the appraisers submit a confidential report to the Magnet Program Office, and this report is then forwarded to the Commission on Magnet Recognition (COM). The Commission members receive "blind" reports to review, and neither the names of the appraiser nor the organization are on the documents (Urden & Monarch, 2002). This final report is reviewed by all members of the Commission, and the decision to award Magnet requires an affirmative vote of two-thirds of the Commission (Urden & Monarch, 2002). The chairperson of the Commission notifies the organization of the decision.

When the CNE receives the call, the formal announcement is made within the organization. Typically, organizations have celebration receptions, buy recognition pins or gifts for all employees, and publish the information in their local newspaper. This is a time to celebrate and to be proud of your achievements. Magnitude of the celebration events varies, and in some organizations, board members and community leaders are invited to the reception.

When Mount Sinai Medical Center in Miami Beach became the 31st hospital awarded Magnet recognition, they were privileged to receive a proclamation from Governor Jeb Bush recognizing their achievement and were honored to have Dan Gelber, a member of the Florida House of Representatives, speak at their ceremony (Messmer, 2001). In addition, the hospital held a "pinning ceremony," in which all the RNs received a Magnet "Excellence in Nursing Service" pin. These pins are available for purchase through the ANCC.

Remember to celebrate and advertise. The organization also receives a Magnet plaque and obelisk, which should be displayed for all patients, visitors, and employees to see.

References

American Nurses Credentialing Center (2003). *The Magnet nursing services recognition program for excellence in nursing service, health care organization, instructions and application process manual (2003–2004 Edition)*. Washington, DC: American Nurses Credentialing Center.

Messmer, P. (2001). Mount Sinai medical center nursing department receives Magnet excellence in nursing services award. *Vital Signs*, June 26, 2001.

Romano, M. (2002). A strong attraction. *Modern Healthcare*, December 16, 2002.

Urden, L., & Monarch, K. (2002). The ANCC Magnet recognition program: Converting research findings into action. In M. McClure & A. Hinshaw (Eds.), *Magnet hospitals revisited: Attraction and retention of professional nurses* (pp. 103–115). Washington, DC: American Nurses Publishing.

Maintaining Magnet status and visibility

Organizational transformation

The celebration is over and everyone who helped the organization obtain Magnet has been recognized for their accomplishments. Now is the time for the team to relax, reflect, and refine. Relaxation is personal but important. Then, after everyone has relaxed, reflection can take place.

A brainstorming retreat away from the hospital offers an opportunity for reflection. Members of the team can discuss the following questions:

- What went well?
- What did employees experience during the process?
- How did we grow as a group and as an organization?
- How do we wish to share this information with our professional colleagues?
- What lessons did we learn?
- What suggestions for improvement did the appraisers share with us?

It is a good idea to keep this activity fun and creative, allowing everyone to reflect on the process.

After the reflective session, come together a second time to refine ideas generated in the brainstorming session. Take this opportunity to discuss the following:

- How do we sustain the positive energy that is flowing through the organization?
- How do we address weaknesses identified during the process?
- Do we need additional resources to sustain the organizational transformation?
- How will we maintain the visibility of our Magnet recognition?
- What organizational changes do we need to make in terms of redesignation?

Begin tackling the issue of recertification from the day of designation—do not wait. "Use Magnet as an ongoing force." Always consider how to make Magnet a vibrant part of a facility's policies and standards.

—Jane Shivnan, MScN, RN, AOCN

The redesignation process should be a day-to-day and annual process in which the facility continually works toward internal improvements. The appraisers look for development —they ask, "what have you changed?" Documentation for redesignation should reflect changes made since the last designation that offer evidence of development over time.

—Toni Fiore, MA, RN,CNAA

Once your organization has achieved Magnet recognition, maintain this visibility in the community. The following key points will prove useful:

- Identify your organization as a Magnet facility in every advertisement published in your local newspaper, nursing journal advertisements, or recruitment brochures
- Revise all hospital brochures/educational material in a timely fashion to reflect Magnet status
- Display a banner at job fairs
- If you have not already done so, notify the deans of your local nursing schools/colleges
- Continually update your hospital and nursing Web site with stories ("Magnet moments") from employees sharing what Magnet means to them and what it is like to work in a Magnet hospital
- Present at local, regional, and national conferences
- Increase membership in and networking with professional organizations
- Publish

One of the most difficult responsibilities of being a Magnet organization is finding the balance between sharing your experiences with organizations just starting the process and not feeling overwhelmed or exhausted by doing so. Some organizations have received as many as one hundred calls from individuals requesting information, seeking tips on the "nitty-gritty" details or asking to come for a site visit. This can be a difficult experience for chief nurse executives (CNE)/Magnet project coordinators: They want to help, but at the same time, it may not be possible to accommodate all the requests. Some ways to share information and minimize the involvement include the following:

- Be a mentor to a select few organizations. Then, as they move along in the process, consider taking on others.
- Hold a partial-day workshop at your facility to share your experiences with a number of individuals at the same time.
- Schedule in advance three or four dates during the year that work for your schedule. Invite multiple individuals to come for a site visit to review documents only on those days.
- Consider posting answers to frequently asked questions on your Web site.
- Dedicate a spot on your Web site to "Magnet memories." Highlight key strategies that were part of your process. You may be able to answer many questions by referring individuals there.

> Responding to e-mails and student requests for assistance with projects about Magnet requires time and resources, so setting up a response system is critical.
>
> **—Laura Caramanica, RN, PhD**

The journey continues

Magnet recognition is awarded for four years, and the organization must comply continually with the program standards, expectations, and eligibility requirements to maintain this status. Magnet hospitals are closely monitored to ensure that they continue to adhere to the rigorous standards; in fact, two hospitals have had their Magnet status revoked (Romano, 2002). The following is a list of changes of which the Magnet organization must inform the Magnet Program Office, in writing, within seven business days of the change:

- Change of chief nursing officer
- Change of medical director
- Change of chief executive officer
- Change in ownership

- Change in profit or nonprofit status
- Sentinel events that potentially compromise patient/resident/client safety or quality of care
- Planned reduction in force
- Any indication of potential instability
- Any information that potentially compromises the ability of the Magnet organization to meet program standards

(From *The Magnet recognition program: Recognizing excellence in nursing services, application manual [2005 Edition].*)

According to the ANCC (2003), an organization may have its Magnet status revoked for failure to notify the Magnet Program Office of any of the above changes, failure to respond to requests for information from the Magnet Program Office in a timely manner, or failure to provide evidence that standards, criteria, and expectations continue to be met.

Over the next four years, Magnet organizations must continue to submit data to the National Database of Nurse Quality Indicators (NDNQI) and provide annual documentation to the Magnet Program Office. The requested information includes the following:

- Hospital demographic data
    - Number of licensed beds
    - Number of staffed beds
    - Average length-of-stay (LOS) for Medicare
    - Average LOS for all payers
- Detailed demographic data
    - Number of registered nurses (RN), including staff, managers, and advanced practice nurses (APN)
    - Number of support staff and unlicensed assistive personnel
    - Number of certified RNs
    - Educational level of staff, including RNs, managers, and APNs
- Vacancy rate, turnover, and termination by unit and job category
- Staffing ratios

- Use of agency nurses
- Use of mandatory overtime
- Average length of RN employment, by unit
- Quality data (NDNQI) results, including trends and interventions
- Results of patient and nurse satisfaction surveys, including trends and interventions

"As of 2004, the redesignation process is the same as the initial process, so the workload is huge. Remember that the Magnet project coordinator position is not a one-time job. Even after recognition is granted, coordinators must process annual reports and coordinate the redesignation effort."

—*Elaine Graf, RN, PhD*

When the documents are submitted, it's important to have a strong infrastructure securely in place to ensure the maintenance of the Magnet standards. An organization that hopes to encourage a Magnet culture should employ a visionary and energetic CNE, skilled nursing leadership, and staff nurses who truly believe in the forces of magnetism and are committed to providing quality care.

—*Kim Sharkey, RN, MBA, CNAA, BC*

When applying for redesignation, "maintain what you have and build onto those." Also, stay abreast of the Magnet requirements as they are revised periodically.

—*Patricia Collins, RN, MSN, AOCN*

When thinking about recertification, remember that the standards are revised every two years, so a facility must stay abreast of any changes made to the standards when reapplying for recognition.

—*Katherine Riley, BSN, RN*

Redesignation

The redesignation process is the same as the original application process including submission of written documents and a site visit. If the eligibility criteria or standards change over the four years, the organization must comply with the new requirements to achieve redesignation. The appraisal fee and site-visit fee are still assessed. The organization must verify the fee structure in place at the time of redesignation.

The good news is that because of ongoing monitoring and your submission of required data, a lot of the work is already in place and complete for redesignation. Committees or councils will have been in place for at least five to six years and will have an abundance of practice examples for the written narratives. To date, all organizations that have obtained Magnet status have had successful redesignations (Urden & Monarch, 2002).

Figure 9.1 is an example of the redesignation timeline from Fox Chase Cancer Center in Philadelphia.

Effective January 2005, organizations need to provide evidence of involvement in community participation and mentoring activities over the past three years.

Figure 9.1 | **Redesignation timeline**

Document	Person responsible	Due date
1. Magnet interim report data due	Magnet Project Coordinator, administrative assistant, Nursing informatics coordinator, nursing financial analyst	July 18, 2003
2. Magnet interim report due to ANCC	Magnet Project Coordinator, administrative assistant	August 10, 2003
3. Order application binders (four full sets: one to ANCC, two for appraisers, one for FCCC) note: Limit four 3-inch binders for each set + one cross reference binder = 20 total needed	Administrative assistant	August 2003
4. Prepare binder tabs, table of contents, cover sheets for each set	Administrative assistant	September 2003
5. Magnet redesignation form/fee	Magnet Project Coordinator, administrative assistant	September 2003
6. Drafts: Standards of care	Section chairs/committee members	August 2003
7. Draft of organizational overview	Members of senior administration	September 2003
8. Drafts: Standards of professional performance	Section chairs/committee members	October 2003
9. Narratives for standards of care	Magnet Project Coordinator	September 2003
10. Narratives for standards of professional performance	Magnet Project Coordinator	November 2003

Figure 9.1

Redesignation timeline (cont.)

Document	Person responsible	Due date
11. Final edit for standards of care section • a unique service emerges that would make coverage determinations inconsistent without clear guidelines	VP nursing/director of nursing research	October 2003
12. Final edit of organizational overview section	Magnet Project Coordinator	November 2003
13. Final edit for standards of professional performance	VP nursing/Director of nursing research	December 2003
14. Application preparation (copies, assembly, binding)	Administrative assistant	December 12, 2003
15. Mail application, appraisal fee, appraisal honorariums	Administrative assistant	January 2004
16. Public notice of application	Administrative assistant, Magnet Project Coordinator	
17. Wait to hear about application, supplemental data		
18. Site visit notification		

Note: Use July 1, 2002, through June 30, 2003, demographic data, acuity data, and staffing data (same as interim report)

Exhibits: Clean, first-print copy

For project data or supporting evidence, use anything after July 1, 2002

Source: Anne Jadwin, Fox Chase Cancer Center in Philadelphia. Reprinted with permission.

References

American Nurses Credentialing Center (2003). *The Magnet nursing services recognition program for excellence in nursing service, health care organization, instructions and application process manual (2003–2004 Edition)*. Washington, DC: American Nurses Credentialing Center.

American Nurses Credentialing Center (2004). *The Magnet recognition program: Recognizing excellence in nursing services application manual (2005 Edition)*. Washington, DC: American Nurses Credentialing Center.

Romano, M. (2002). A strong attraction. *Modern Healthcare*, December 16, 2002.

Urden, L., & Monarch, K. (2002). The ANCC Magnet recognition program: Converting research findings into action. In M. McClure & A. Hinshaw (Eds.), *Magnet hospitals revisited: Attraction and retention of professional nurses* (pp. 103–115). Washington, DC: American Nurses Publishing.

Integration of nursing research

By Susan H. Nick, RN, PhD, independent consultant

The Magnet Recognition Program requires that the chief nurse executive (CNE) support research and integrate it into the delivery of nursing care and nursing administration. This is achieved by identifying contemporary practice issues to be studied, reviewing proposed research studies, ensuring protection of human subjects, using research findings in clinical practice, and identifying resources needed to support research projects. In this chapter, you will learn about components of a nursing research program, learn how to incorporate evidence-based practice into day-to-day operations, learn how nursing research connects to the institutional review board (IRB), and discuss the differences between quality improvement and research.

Questions to be asked in assessing the organization's research readiness for Magnet include the following.

| Figure 10.1 | Research readiness checklist |

Question	Yes	No
Are nurses involved in clinical and administrative investigations that have been identified using the nursing process?		
Are nurses rewarded for participating in nursing research studies?		
Are processes in place for nurses to report on the results of nursing research?		
Does the facility have a library with the resources to support nursing research?		
Are the nursing policies and procedures based on evidence-based practices?		
Do faculty from local colleges and universities collaborate with nursing staff on research projects?		
Is there a nursing research committee in place?		
Is nursing represented on the organization's institutional review board (IRB)?		
Are educational programs in place to assist nurses with the nursing research process and the research utilization process?		
Does the organization subscribe to an online evidence-based practice Web site?		
Are there advanced practice nurses (APN) to support the research process?		
Do all nurses have access to the Internet?		

Evidenced-based practice

Nurses want to provide the best care for their patients. However, nurses often rely on clinical experiences, traditions, and untested actions to carry out their responsibilities. Evidenced-based practice relies on research findings, quality improvement data, other evaluation data, and the consensus of recognized experts for substantiation. It expects that nurses will always question why they do things and look for better ways of achieving goals. This kind of practice has been shown to improve care, with 28% better outcomes than those of control patients reported in a meta analysis by Heater (1988).

Nurses often cite lack of time and staffing shortages as the reasons they do not investigate practice databases. But another reason is lack of education about the research process and the utilization process. In order for nurses to recognize the importance of evidenced-based practice, they must be supported by the nursing leaders. The CNE can champion an environment in which research findings are used to improve nursing practice. This is achieved through selected activities that include the following:

- Hiring a doctoral- or master's-prepared nurse to enhance staff's understanding of evidence-based practice
- Developing an awareness campaign
- Partnering with a local university for its faculty expertise
- Initiating a nursing research committee
- Inviting expert speakers to present examples of evidence-based practice
- Sponsoring a nurse to become a research nurse intern within the organization or at another hospital with such a program
- Including nursing research involvement in the steps of a clinical ladder
- Including evidence-based practice expectations in all nursing job descriptions, including that of the CNE
- Hiring nurses who are interested in working in an organization that values improving care through evidence-based practice or nurses who are open to learning about new ways of practicing
- Conducting journal club activities with nurses at all levels of the organization
- Developing a structured critique worksheet to rate the quality of evidence and the benefits and feasibility of using the findings in the organization's practice (Agency for Healthcare Research and Quality—AHRQ—has a rating scale for research reviews)

- Accessing the Grateful Med Web site to use Medline for literature searches

- Evaluating practice and then reevaluating whenever changes are made

- Developing a recognition program for nurses involved in evidence-based practice (Nurses' Week is a good time to present this recognition program)

Common barriers

Recognize the barriers to implementing evidence-based practice in your organization and prepare an action plan to address them. Some barriers that may exist in your organization include the following:

- Staff nurses have little control over their workload

- Hospitals rely on overtime hours for patient care

- Hospital mergers mix divergent cultures

- Some nurses don't recognize the need to change their practice

- There is a lack of support from administration

- Many nurses lack training in effective literature searching and research methodology

When implementing changes in a large organization, consider conducting a pilot demonstration of the change on one or two units. During the pilot, obtain feedback from staff and management to adapt, adopt, or reject the changes. Once the changes work smoothly, they can be rolled out on additional units.

The advanced practice nurses (APN) are best educated to lead the movement to evidence-based practice. They also have the clinical expertise to develop protocols specific to patient populations. The CNE who champions this effort should meet with the APNs on a regular basis—at least quarterly—to monitor progress and ensure that the APNs have the resources they need to implement evidence-based practice. This group of nurses can participate in activities that encourage others to learn more about evidence-based practice, by

- pursuing research projects
- presenting lectures in the hospital and at regional and national conferences
- leading support groups
- covering for staff who are attending evidence-based practice meetings or journal clubs
- tracking practice changes in the literature

- monitoring compliance with new protocols
- reeducating staff about protocols
- helping staff to initiate evidence-based practice projects
- seeking grant funding for evidence-based practice projects; look to national nursing organizations, philanthropic support, and the federal government as potential funding sources

Examples of evidence-based practice projects

- Have staff manage the confused hospitalized elderly patient
- Discuss how to determine whether chlorhexidine is a more effective skin antiseptic than other cleansing agents in preventing probable peripheral intravenous catheter-related infection
- Develop an orientation brochure on hospitalization for patients and families, and monitor its effect on patient satisfaction
- Evaluate an inservice intervention aimed at increasing the use of alternatives to restraints
- Assess adequacy of pain treatment in first 24 hours postoperatively
- Determine how you can promote smoking cessation

Establishing a nursing research committee

A nursing research committee (NRC) allows for a larger group—not just the nursing research coordinator—to be involved in the process. Often these committees are multidisciplinary and include physicians, pharmacists, and other clinicians as well as staff nurses, nurse managers, quality improvement coordinators, nurse educators, and APNs. This interdisciplinary, hospital-wide committee sets goals around the research process. These goals may include

- suggesting improvement projects
- coordinating journal clubs
- sponsoring research symposia
- providing education to staff about both the research process and utilization of best practices
- hosting research poster/paper presentation sessions
- assisting with development of research studies
- facilitating work with a biostatistician
- evaluating/approving research proposals
- providing a liaison to IRB

- contributing to nursing newsletter
- working with policy and procedure committee to develop evidence-based standards and policies
- presenting research awards

Although staff nurses often are reluctant, initially, to participate in nursing research projects, the presence of a nursing research committee can help to ensure project completion. Therefore, members of the committee should be committed to nursing research. Other success factors include

- regularly scheduled meetings, so that members do not forget when they are
- a high level of research expertise across the committee
- familiarity with the IRB process
- a diverse representation of expertise
- an understanding of the "forming, storming, and norming" steps of group development

Some organizations have unit-based committees in addition to hospital-wide NRCs. This committee works with staff to initiate evidence-based practice studies specific to the population of patients on their unit. It also chooses journal articles pertinent to their practice. The hospital-wide NRC is responsible for ensuring the standardization of evidence-based practice across the organization. This oversight also prevents duplication of efforts in the unit-based committees and assists with collaboration of the committees.

Unit-based committees actually conduct group projects and use them to draw interested staff nurses into the research process. Committee members must understand that everyone's role is important and contributes to the success of the project. Members of the unit-based committees also can identify specific tasks in the research process and divide them among themselves. Some tasks will require more than one person to complete and thus can be assigned to a small group. Tasks include

- coordinating the project
- identifying the problem
- literature search and analysis
- selecting a research design
- preparing the protocol for the review process

- collecting data
- analyzing data or working with a biostatistician
- writing reports
- identifying how practice will change
- disseminating findings in articles, newsletters, and presentations

Journal clubs

Journal clubs introduce staff nurses to research, and the articles reviewed can be used to support evidence-based practice initiatives. Additionally, the articles can serve as the beginning review of the literature for publications of research studies.

An important first step is the identification of journal articles for discussion. Journal clubs can take a number of different forms. You can have article discussions as part of a standing meeting, in a separate meeting, in an online chatroom, or as an electronic listserv. The journal club can be interdisciplinary with a focus on nursing practice. Here are some guidelines for a journal club that Dr. Turkel and I have found to be useful in the practice setting:

- First, identify journal articles to discuss. Internet access makes literature searches easy for staff. The Internet can be used to find articles and evidence-based practice information. Government Web sites are free to individuals using them, while other Web sites may have fees for access to member-only sections. Examples of available Web sites follow.

Figure 10.2 **Evidence-based practice Web sites**

Organization	Web Site	Description
Agency for Healthcare Research and Quality	www.ahrq.gov	Government agency offering information about evidence-based practice for all disciplines
Canadian Centre for Health Evidence	www.cche.net	Canadian agency promoting evidence-based practice
National Guideline Clearinghouse	www.guideline.gov	Several organizations have partnered to offer a comprehensive database of evidence-based clinical practice guidelines
National Library of Medicine	www.nlm.nih.gov	A site to search for evidence-based practice information
Evidence-Based Nursing	www.ebn.bmjjournals.com	Web site for evidence-based nursing journal
Sarah Cole Hirsh Institute for Best Nursing Practices Based on Evidence	http://fpb.cwru.edu/HirshInstitute	The Frances Payne Bolton School of Nursing at Case Western Reserve University site offers reviews, conferences, and consulting services

Each nursing unit or division must decide how to conduct its journal article review. If the review will occur during a meeting, identify a standing time and location. Meetings can be "on the go" for 15 minutes, with rotating participants, or can last longer with more in-depth discussion.

Once that's decided, identify a facilitator for the meeting. Initially, this person should be a nurse with either a masters degree or a bachelors degree, but, as all members of the nursing staff become more comfortable with the process, the role of facilitator should be rotated among all participants.

Prior to the meeting, the facilitator distributes the article to be discussed (preferably, leaving two weeks for staff to read it). He or she should leave copies in the nursing lounge and in the individual mailboxes of nurses interested in participating. All participants will be responsible for reading the article and performing their own critique of the article (provide a form/checklist for this critique).

In the meeting, have fun and encourage participation. Focus the discussion on the relevance of the content to nursing practice. If the discussion is electronic, the facilitator is responsible for initiating the dialogue with a brief abstract of the article and some questions to stimulate a critique. Ask participants to "reply all" when responding so everyone has the benefit of reading what their peers have to say about the article. Keep the discussion open for a three-week time period and then summarize its key points.

After the meeting, evaluate the journal club discussion (including the role of the facilitator, how many nurses participated, whether they were able to discuss the article, whether they could identify relevance to practice, etc.). The facilitator must keep the signed attendance sheet or the electronic discussion and a copy of the article in the unit-based nursing research binder.

Then, share the articles with members of the hospital-wide research committee to be used on other nursing units, if appropriate, and decide the club's next step based on the discussion (e.g., read another article on the same topic, change a protocol or policy, suggest changes to administration, make no changes, etc.).

Collaboration with hospital IRB

The IRB consists of a multidisciplinary group of individuals from an institution who review proposed and ongoing research for the purpose of protecting human subjects. In addition to hospital or organizational personnel, members of the IRB include community members. If the organization receives any federal funds to pay for research, the IRB will follow strict federal guidelines for reviewing proposals, but whether federally funded or not, investigators must ensure that their research plans are ethical. The IRB provides external review for the investigator to eliminate any researcher biases in determining the ethics of the project.

The NRC must know the policies of its organization's IRB. When preparing protocol for a specific study, members should review all IRB forms to be completed and ensure that they are signed by the appropriate administrators and investigators. The IRB committee should include nursing representation so nurses can keep up to date on how protocols impact workflow and what resources are required to carry out the protocols on nursing units. The quality improvement coordinator, research nurse, nurse educators, and APNs could serve as representatives to the IRB.

One of the primary ethical considerations in research involving human subjects is informed consent, which ensures that subjects understand the research study and voluntarily agree to participate in it. The consent form must be written in understandable language, preferably at the sixth grade level, and should avoid or explain technical or medical terms. Consents can be written or oral, based on the policies of your organizations IRB. There are times when the consent is waived, again based on the organization's IRB policies.

The written consent form should include the following elements:

- A statement that the study involves research
- An explanation of the purposes of the research
- The expected duration of the subject's participation
- A description of the procedures to be followed
- Identification of any procedures that are experimental
- A description of any foreseeable risks/discomforts to subjects
- A description of any benefits to the subjects
- A disclosure of alternative procedures or courses of treatment
- A statement explaining confidentiality of records
- A statement about compensation, if any
- An explanation as to whether any medical treatments are available if injury occurs due to the research

- A contact person for answers to questions about the research and the research process
- A statement that participation in the research is voluntary
- A statement that care and benefits are available if the subject declines to participate in the research
- A statement that the participant may discontinue participation at any time without any penalties or breaks in treatment
- A statement that the subject will be given a copy of the consent
- A place for the subject's signature (or, in the case of a minor, a place for the guardian to sign and the child to give assent)

The IRB is responsible for making sure that the risks of a research protocol are reasonable in relation to the potential benefits of the study. The IRB realizes there might not be any benefits for the individual participant but wants to know that there could be future benefits. Sometimes the nurses are concerned about this external review of their protocol, but when put in the perspective of protecting human subjects, it should be an easier process.

Research v. quality improvement

Clinicians are often unsure of the difference between research and quality improvement activities. It is an important distinction because research projects require the approval of the IRB and quality improvement projects do not.

Research is defined by Department of Health and Human Services (HHS) regulations as systematic investigation—including development, testing and/or evaluation—designed to develop or contribute to generalizable knowledge. In the context of these issues, generalizable knowledge is held to be knowledge related to health that can be applied to populations outside the population being studied. That is, participants in a research project may or may not benefit directly from the study, but a larger group is expected to gain from the knowledge obtained in the study. The investigator conducting research uses a randomized sample and normally intends to publish the results in a scientific journal.

In its August 2001 document, Ethical and Policy Issues in Research Involving Human Subjects, the National Bioethics Advisory Commission (NBAC) explains quality improvement activities as those in the health services area not intended to generate scientific knowledge but rather used as a management tool to improve the provision of services to a specific healthcare population. These activities are not intended to have any application outside the specific organization in which they are conducted.

Quality-improvement projects used to analyze and improve hospital operations do not qualify as research and do not need to be reviewed by the IRB. However, if a quality-improvement project is undertaken with the intent of publishing the results or presenting the results in a setting outside the organization, then it should be considered research and be reviewed by the IRB.

Also differentiate between quality improvement and quality assurance. In a study by Bottrell (2003), quality-improvement coordinators identified quality assurance as retrospective record review to measure that a particular activity is happening within agreed-upon parameters. The same group of coordinators thought quality improvement went beyond that to examine different ways of practicing and to determine what is better with known and accepted modes of treatment.

But ethical considerations arise in quality improvement as well as in research. The research process includes IRB or external review process. An organization should consider creating an oversight committee to review the ethics of quality-improvement activities before undertaking them. This administrative review would ensure that all the Health Insurance Portability and Accountability Act (HIPAA) regulations for confidentiality are upheld.

Both quality improvement and research projects can be used to develop evidence-based practice protocols. No matter which source is used, once implemented, the protocol needs to be evaluated and perhaps modified with continual improvements.

Summary

In order to achieve Magnet recognition, the organization must be able to demonstrate that nursing care is based on evidence-based practice, which includes conducting research, utilizing research results, and identifying practice problems through the quality-improvement process, the research process, patient-satisfaction data, focus groups, or discussions with staff. The CNE must be the champion of this initiative. In addition, master's- and bachelor's-prepared nurses provide unit-based leadership for evidence-based practice. Partnering with local colleges and universities helps to increase the number of master's-prepared nurses working on evidence-based practice initiatives. The purpose of initiating evidence-based practice is to improve patient outcomes.

References

Bottrell, M. (July, 2003). "The ethics of quality improvement: Practitioners' perspectives." Paper presented to Veteran's Health Administration, National Center for Ethics in Health Care, San Francisco.

Heater, B. (1988). Nursing intervention and patient outcomes: A meta-analysis of studies. *Nursing Research*, 37(5), 303–307.

Kohn, L., Corrigan, J., Donaldson, M. (Eds.) (2000). *To err is human: Building a safer health care system*. Washington, DC: National Academy Press.

National Bioethics Advisory Commission (2001). *Ethical and policy issues in research involving human participants (Volume I)*. Bethesda, MD: Government Printing Office.

Best practices and lessons learned along the way

Introduction

Now that you have decided to embark on the Magnet journey, I would like to share with you some of the ideas, thoughts, and practice examples from your peers who have successfully obtained Magnet status in their organization, are currently in the middle of the application process, or recently had a successful recertification of their Magnet status. They will provide you with an opportunity to learn and benefit from others' experiences. Networking and collaboration are important for organizations to create and sustain professional and positive work environments, and I hope these examples assist you as you begin the cultural transformation and Magnet process in your organization.

I was unable to include best practices from all Magnet facilities, but there are many overlapping themes in the following examples, which is how the chapter is organized. Remember, some ideas may be perfect for your organization and others may not be as useful. I tried to cover the full spectrum of the Magnet experience through these examples. I am thankful to all of the chief nurse executives or Magnet coordinators who took time from their busy schedules to contribute to this chapter. Some of the quotes are direct and some are paraphrased. All the comments are all excellent and they are not arranged in order of importance. All of them are valuable, and I want to thank these leaders for being advocates not only for their nursing staff but for all professional nurses.

Embarking on the journey for the right reasons

"The primary purpose should be altruistic." That is, facilities should achieve recognition because "facilitating a Magnet culture as a nurse leader is the right thing to do." The standards should drive the creation of the Magnet environment, and you should invest time and effort in the standards because they benefit the nursing staff and, ultimately, patients—not because the board of trustees has requested that Magnet designation be pursued for marketing purposes. Simply put, pursue recognition for the right reasons.

—Kim Hitchings, RN, MSN

Create an organization with point-of-care accountability for decision-making. "The commitment and dedication toward making Saint Joseph's Hospital a place where nurses could work with significant autonomy of professional practice created the infrastructure that supported and sustained a culture of nursing excellence."

—Kim Sharkey, RN, MBA, CNAA, BC

Nursing leadership must be compelled to achieve Magnet status because they want to create a positive work environment for their nurses and, consequently, improve nursing morale, not so they can put a plaque on the wall. Whether there's an award should not matter. The benefits of working at a Magnet facility should convince leadership to begin the journey to achieve Magnet.

—Toni Fiore, MA, RN, CNAA

"One of the best benefits of Magnet recognition is not the award itself, but the environment the award is recognizing." Cultivating an environment in which nurses' work is valued is important regardless of whether an organization pursues Magnet.

—Beverly Hancock, MS, RN

Staying aware of time constraints

Allow enough time. You cannot anticipate how long final approval and editing of the documentation will take before it leaves the institution. It's critical to know who needs to sign off on the materials before they leave the hospital (e.g., legal staff, nursing leadership), and then you must give the appropriate officials ample time to review and approve the documents.

—Jane Shivnan, MScN, RN, AOCN

Aside from securing approval from the necessary people, the coordinator must assemble the final documents, work with the printer, and perform a final edit. It is a meticulous, time-consuming process not unlike publishing a book. It takes time to ensure you are delivering a quality product to the reviewers. Also, pay attention to such minor yet important details as knowing that the final paper is likely to be thicker than standard paper. Committees probably work with standard paper while they're in the draft stage, but the printer typically uses quality paper for the final version. Details like these, while seemingly trivial, can present a roadblock in your timeline if you fail to take them into account.

—*Jane Shivnan, MScN, RN, AOCN*

Facilities must appreciate the immense, organized, and tightly focused effort required to submit documentation. "Pulling it all together was huge."

—*Barbara Wadsworth, RN, MSN, CNAA*

Involving the nursing staff and securing buy-in

Keep the staff engaged. "Celebrate everything."

—*Barbara Wadsworth, RN, MSN, CNAA*

Form a Magnet executive team of interdepartmental system executives. The goal of this team is to determine how to best support nursing to achieve Magnet designation. Keep them informed about your progress toward Magnet and they will keep their departments informed.

—*Norine Watson, RN, MSN, CNA, BC*

Engage the staff from the beginning. Solicit feedback from the nursing staff about why they feel they are a Magnet facility. This allows them to identify what they're most proud of in their work on the units.

—*Elaine Graf, RN, PhD*

Involve everyone in the journey, from housekeepers to dietitians, and clerks to nursing assistants. "Nursing does not exist in a vacuum and it takes everyone to create a climate of nursing excellence. We gave everyone our Magnet buttons, which we designed for our own initiative, and everyone wore them to signify their support. After we achieved our Magnet award, we gave out Magnet pins to everyone from administrators to housekeepers (those connected with nursing units who were identified by nurses as people integral to their success as caregivers) in recognition of their support of nursing and their support of the Magnet initiative."

—Barbara Hannon, MSN, RN

After each cycle, assess what worked and what didn't and implement changes. Use a shared governance professional practice model to involve staff in the process.

—Kim Sharkey, RN, MBA, CNAA, BC

Communicating

Enlist a communication committee to assist in communication efforts, ranging from articles in newsletters, educational offerings (a traveling learning board), games, and contests.

—Janice Mains, RN, MS

Make sure Magnet is an agenda item at every meeting.

—Barbara Wadsworth, RN, MSN, CNAA

Host a Magnet cover design contest in which members from anywhere in the facility can compete to create the application's cover.

—Anne Jadwin, RN, MSN, AOCN, CNA

Create an internal newsletter and use it as a vehicle to keep staff informed of all Magnet issues. Communication is key.

—Toni Fiore, MA, RN, CNAA

Include articles in the medical staff newsletter highlighting the value of pursuing Magnet and how achieving recognition will positively impact physicians. Present educational overviews of the Magnet program to physicians and other medical staff leadership.

—Cole Edmonson, MS, RN, CHE, CNAA, BC

Offer a Magnet inservice for every department. Develop a teaching manual of the key Magnet standards and distribute it to every hospital department. At unit staff meetings, discuss how

Magnet recognition will benefit the facility. Communicate with all stakeholders throughout the process.

—Janet Wright, MSN, RN, BC

Maintain dialogue among various departments within the organization throughout the Magnet journey. Use newsletters, e-mails, and meetings to communicate with staff on all shifts about Magnet.

—Janet Ahlstrom, MSN, RN, BC, M-SCNS

Defining the committee structure

Johns Hopkins used two committees for the two different phases of the project. One committee was the Magnet advisory council with representation from all areas. This was a nurse leadership group that met for a half hour every week for four months, tackled the standards, and brainstormed ideas for the written portion of the documentation.

—Jane Shivnan, MScN, RN, AOCN

Children's Memorial Medical Center created a nursing quality council within their shared governance structure. All units were represented. "They became the foundation to all quality initiatives and had a direct reporting relationship to our hospital quality board." The Magnet steering committee at Children's Memorial Medical Center originally met monthly, but at each meeting little had been accomplished. Changing to weekly meetings moved the process along more quickly and made Magnet written documentation a higher priority for all involved.

—Elaine Graf, RN, PhD

The team must include computer-savvy, bright, and energetic people who are willing to work long hours if necessary. If possible, use technical assistants to set up meetings, gather information, take pictures, and organize any attachments.

—Patricia Collins, RN, MSN, AOCN

Begin with a top-down philosophy (in which the person who led the Magnet initiative first meets with board members and executive staff to connect the realities of the facility to the Magnet standards) and let it evolve to leaders at the bedside.

—Toni Fiore, MA, RN, CNAA

Assign the standards to the appropriate staff within the facility with timelines and specific instructions on what the facility requires for evidence of compliance.

—Cole Edmonson, MS, RN, CHE, CNAA, BC

Selecting ambassadors and Magnet champions

Appoint Magnet champions who are also staff nurses. They should run the Magnet fair, report back to their units any information on the progress of the project, and choose a theme and logo for the Magnet journey.

—Susan Palette-Gallagher, MA, RN, CNAA, BC

Appoint Magnet ambassadors from the nursing units and other departments within the facility. Keep them updated and ask them for feedback. These ambassadors communicate directly to their units and departments about the Magnet journey. They are the Magnet "cheerleaders." Make sure the meetings with the ambassadors are fun.

—Patricia Collins, RN, MSN, AOCN

Have nurse managers identify champions or ambassadors from each unit. Provide an off-site training day in which they receive information that they can relay back to their colleagues. Staff nurses must be fully involved every step of the way. They are especially critical to the site visit.

—Toni Fiore, MA, RN, CNAA

Writing the narrative

A smaller writing team can lead to greater success. Employing many people to generate ideas is smart, but it's helpful to have only a few people actually involved in the writing process. Stay organized around the writing and have an editor coordinate the writing process.

—Suzanne Beyea, RN, PhD, FAAN

Designate sufficient time to spend on writing the narratives. Stick to tackling narratives for no more than two standards in one day.

—Anne Jadwin, RN, MSN, AOCN, CNA

Create a shared drive in the facility's computer system that can only be accessed by the writers of the documentation and the technical assistants. This creates an opportunity for peer review, ensures consistency, and reduces redundancy.

—Patricia Collins, RN, MSN, AOCN

When organizing materials to be included in the documentation, focus on examples of creativity and innovation within the facility.

—Patricia Collins, RN, MSN, AOCN

The writers should meet with the CNO on a regular basis to solicit feedback and recommendations on the documentation.

—Patricia Collins, RN, MSN, AOCN

In the final stages of the narrative, meet once or twice a week and showcase the documentation on an overhead so that everyone in the meeting can critique and improve the written work. This type of peer review is invaluable. "It really brought a sense of enthusiasm as we shared collectively what we individually compiled."

—Deborah Ford, RN, BSN, MSN, CNA

Keep the documentation writing team small (five to six people in the beginning stages with one person in charge as the work is finalized). Too many voices cloud the clarity of the document.

—Toni Fiore, MA, RN, CNAA

"It is very important to take the standards in draft form to the staff nurses. We had about 80 staff nurse Magnet champions representing every inpatient and outpatient unit in our hospital. I took all the drafts of the standards to them and spent one afternoon with them critiquing the proposed versions. The staff nurses told the Magnet Steering Committee that we were missing some great nursing programs, projects, and innovative practices, so I went back to the drawing board and rewrote probably 40% of the standards using the ideas and suggestions from those nurses closest to the patients, the staff nurses. So a word of advice is that having all the standards written by nursing management will create a deficit of information about actual bedside practices. Therefore, including staff nurses in the process is critical."

—*Barbara Hannon, MSN, RN*

"It is extremely important to create databases of evidence and assign certain programs and pieces of evidence to certain standards so that the same data is not used by two people as an example to clarify two separate standards."

—*Barbara Hannon, MSN, RN*

Host open forums on all units to solicit feedback and stories about how the hospital meets the Magnet standards so that the narrative is a reflection of everyone's input.

—*Laura Caramanica, RN, PhD*

Invite staff nurses to sit in on committee meetings as the Magnet team writes documents and plans communication strategies.

—*Janis Mains, RN, MS*

The written portion of the application was the most time intensive and took nine months to complete.

—*Cole Edmonson, MS, RN, CHE, CNAA, BC*

Gathering/submitting data

Gathering the demographic data, although cumbersome, is critical so that nursing leadership can make important decisions about hiring and continuing education.

—*Elaine Graf, RN, PhD*

"Build the 'fields' that you need to complete for ANA Report Card in your collection tools/systems so that you don't have to do chart reviews for data and so that it is as seamless as possible. We are working on our plan for our automated medical record to try to capture all quality data so that the labor intensive process of auditing charts is as small as it needs to be. Have clinicians drive this process and have them see this as important feedback. Hold staff and managers accountable for the outcomes in performance reviews."

—Laura Caramanica, RN, PhD

Conduct an RN survey using the ANA tool on the years you do not conduct an RN survey using the HR tool. Look at the data from the employee survey. Analyze different segments of the staff separately and compare it to data from other years. Most importantly, *act on the data*. Talk with your staff about the results. There are often discrepancies between what you meant when asking the questions and what respondents meant when answering them. Don't make assumptions. To get this feedback, conduct a round-the-clock open forum in every shift (although it may take months, it's well worth the time).

—Laura Caramanica, RN, PhD

In earlier years, Hartford Hospital had difficulty obtaining meaningful data as defined by ANA database requirements because its systems were not set up to collect the data. Over the years, it's changed its collection process so it can work with a system that collects the required data as defined by ANA (e.g., its automated incident report system collects all questions asked on the fall data sheet) to cut down on labor-intensive chart reviews. The staff collects data and provides reports for both the Magnet project and all other reporting agencies. Fulfilling annual data requirements and ensuring accuracy and timeliness of reporting puts a strain on resources and staff. "This is, however, what it takes to participate."

—Laura Caramanica, RN, PhD

"At one time, we had no idea how many of our nurses were certified in their specialties, volunteering in the community, or attending college classes. We created an Excel spreadsheet listing all nurses for each unit and asked the manager (or their designee) to keep it up-to-date. Now this information is easily obtainable."

—Patricia Collins, RN, MSN, AOCN

Nursing at Johns Hopkins works well with human resources (HR) in part because of an HR representative who jointly reports to both HR and the VP of nursing. She or he can work as liaison who focuses on nursing HR and can easily obtain the information requested.

—Jane Shivnan, MScN, RN, AOCN

Identifying the challenges

"One challenge is that when you achieve this designation, you are more visible and your outcome indicators are looked at with closer scrutiny, and you feel you have to be the best in everything you do and that's hard to do every moment."

—*Laura Caramanica, RN, PhD*

Getting 3,000 nurses organized into one focused effort.

—*Norine Watson, RN, MSN, CNA, BC*

A large, busy academic institution like Johns Hopkins faces unique challenges. "Our challenge was balancing the sensitivity to all the different demands on nurse's time and energy with our commitment as an organization to making our Magnet journey meaningful." One goal was to avoid stressing the department of nursing and its resources.

—*Jane Shivnan, MScN, RN, AOCN*

"The biggest challenge in applying for the recognition was to demonstrate compliance with the standards and criterion for nursing research and evidence-based practice. These concepts were not very evident in the service environment and need to be more clearly demonstrated."

—*Cole Edmonson, MS, RN, CHE, CNAA, BC*

"A challenge we had was reporting staffing HR information to Magnet: It was a totally different computation of skill mix, FTE configuration, and hours per patient days. We had to calculate RN vacancy and turnover rates by positions rather than FTE. The ANCC formula is based on FTEs. Because we had not tracked either LPN or PCT turnover or vacancy rates, we did utilize the ANCC formula with FTEs for these."

—*Janis Mains, RN, MS*

Gathering the required quality and demographic data. When Children's Memorial Medical Center began the project, they had just implemented a new scheduling system that also tracked staff credentials, which is what they use to electronically send their yearly updates to ANCC. "As the system improves and ANCC becomes clearer on what they are seeking, it has been smoother. The process is dynamic and, as such, ever changing."

—*Elaine Graf, RN, PhD*

Compiling the immense amount of data and writing the material in an organized, reader-friendly format.

—*Elizabeth Warden, RN, CNA, MS*

"The ongoing challenges are related to the growth and evolution of the program. "Each redesignation has provided us the privilege to use a different manual and a different format for submission of data."

—*Kim Sharkey, RN, MBA, CNAA, BC*

Looking back

Medical City Dallas Hospital and The North Texas Hospital for Children would have pursued Magnet much earlier. "The process was very rewarding as a whole and allowed us an opportunity to look at the details of the nursing service that existed at the organization for improvement."

—*Cole Edmonson, MS, RN, CHE, CNAA, BC*

"It is a constant journey and it will have ups and downs."

—*Laura Caramanica, RN, PhD*

Today, healthcare is a rapidly changing industry. Magnet designation is an incentive to continuously raise the standards of the delivery of optimal patient care. There should be an expectation of continued growth, with a facility building on previous accomplishments and implementing progressive changes for the future.

—*Kim Sharkey, RN, MBA, CNAA, BC*

"Being a Magnet coordinator was the best job in my life."

—*Jane Shivnan, MScN, RN, AOCN*

"Because Magnet recognition is about the culture of the organization, there is always a need to stay focused on that to ensure that the forces of Magnetism are still with you."

—*Katherine Riley, BSN, RN*